Introduction

Rheumatoid arthritis (RA) is the commonest inflammatory joint disease, affecting approximately 1% of adults in the developed world. It may seem surprising, therefore, that what we know about this disease is far outweighed by what we do not. In this text we have attempted to provide a simplified overview of how RA is thought to develop, how it is diagnosed and monitored, and how it is treated. Fortunately, elements of RA pathogenesis are now becoming unravelled and, more than in any other disease, this has led to powerful targeted treatments. These are discussed in the closing chapters of the book, along with our thoughts on future directions of investigation and management.

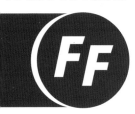

FAST FACTS

Indispensable
Guides to
Clinical
Practice

Rheumatoid Arthritis

John D Isaacs
Reader, Rheumatology and
Rehabilitation Research Unit,
University of Leeds, UK

Larry W Moreland
Director, Arthritis Clinical Intervention Program,
The University of Alabama at Birmingham,
USA

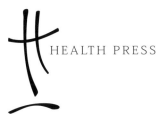

HEALTH PRESS

Oxford

Fast Facts – Rheumatoid Arthritis
First published April 2002

Text © 2002 John D Isaacs, Larry W Moreland
© 2002 in this edition Health Press Limited
Health Press Limited, Elizabeth House, Queen Street, Abingdon,
Oxford OX14 3JR, UK
Tel: +44 (0)1235 523233
Fax: +44 (0)1235 523238

Fast Facts is a trade mark of Health Press Limited.

A CIP catalogue record for this title is available from the British
Library.

ISBN 1-903734-16-9

Isaacs, JD (John D)
Fast Facts – Rheumatoid Arthritis/
John D Isaacs, Larry W Moreland

Printed by Fine Print (Services) Ltd, Oxford, UK.

Glossary of acronyms

ACR: American College of Rheumatology

BRM: biological response modifier

COX: cyclooxygenase

DAS: disease activity score

DEXA: dual emission x-ray absorptiometry

DMARD: disease-modifying anti-rheumatic drug

EMEA: European Agency for the Evaluation of Medical Products

FBC: full blood count (complete blood cell count, CBC, in the USA)

FDA: Food and Drug Administration

HAQ: Stanford Health Assessment Questionnaire

HRUS: high-resolution ultrasound

IL: interleukin

mAb: monoclonal antibody

MAPK: mitogen-activated protein kinase

MCP: metacarpo-phalangeal

MMP: matrix metalloproteinase

MTP: metatarso-phalangeal

NICE: National Institute for Clinical Excellence

NSAID: non-steroidal anti-inflammatory drug

OCIF: osteoclastogenesis inhibitory factor

ODF: osteoclast differentiation factor

RA: rheumatoid arthritis

RhF: rheumatoid factor

TGF: transforming growth factor

TIMP: tissue inhibitor of metalloproteinases

TNF: tumour necrosis factor

Normal synovium

The synovial membrane lines the non-weight-bearing aspects of the synovial cavity (Figure 1.1) and is divided into the lining layer or intima and sub-lining layer or sub-intima.

The intima is just one or two cell layers thick and contains two major cell types: type A synoviocytes, which bear macrophage markers, and type B synoviocytes, which have fibroblastic characteristics. The intima lacks typical features of an epithelium and does not possess a basement membrane or tight intercellular contacts between synoviocytes. The matrix of the intima is rich in proteoglycans and glycosaminoglycans, in particular hyaluronic acid.

The sub-intima is a loose, vascular connective tissue stroma containing blood vessels, lymphatics and nerve endings within a matrix

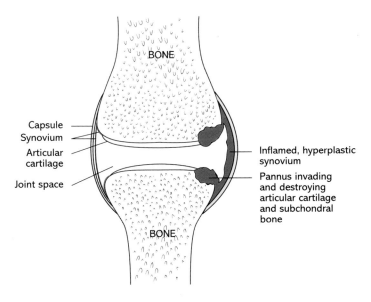

Figure 1.1 Diagrammatic representation of normal joint anatomy (left side of figure) and RA pathology (right).

comprising varying proportions of lipid, collagen fibrils and more organized fibrous tissue.

Synovial fluid

The synovial membrane secretes lubricating and nourishing synovial fluid, a viscous fluid containing a high concentration of hyaluronic acid. Other constituents include nutrients and solutes that diffuse from the blood vessels in the sub-intima. The precise physiology of synovial fluid production is unknown, but exchange of fluid between the circulation and the joint space is governed by a balance of hydrostatic, osmotic and convective forces. As well as providing an osmotic force within the synovial cavity, hyaluronic acid contributes to the lubricating properties of synovial fluid although other, undefined constituents are also important.

Articular cartilage

Articular cartilage comprises chondrocytes embedded in a hydrated matrix composed of collagen, proteoglycans and other matrix proteins. It is an avascular structure lacking lymphatics, and the synovial fluid is critical for providing nutrients to this tissue. Water makes up approximately 70% of normal cartilage by weight, whereas chondrocytes occupy only 5–10% by volume. Because of their low density, chondrocytes do not come into contact with one another directly but possess cellular processes which abut the matrix. These cells are critical to the integrity of articular cartilage because they synthesize collagen, proteoglycans and also other components such as fibronectin. Each cell is surrounded by a zone of secreted proteoglycan and a basket-like mantle of fibrillar collagen, but the highest collagen content occurs in the more distal intercellular matrix.

Collagens are fibrillar proteins that, together with proteoglycans, account for the biomechanical properties of articular cartilage. There are 14 different types of collagen, divided into three major groups. The predominant collagen in articular cartilage is type II, constituting approximately 90% in the adult, with types IX and XI contributing most of the remainder. All collagens are based on a triple helical structure (Figure 1.2), and the differences between collagens relate to either the length of the triple helix, the presence of non-collagenous units within the molecule that impart extra flexibility, or the addition of non-collagenous side-chains such as carbohydrates. The triple helical structure of collagens accounts for their tensile strength. Collagen biosynthetic and degradative pathways are quite well characterized. Quantification of byproducts of collagen II synthesis (procollagen propeptides) and breakdown (collagen cross-links) in synovial fluid or urine have been tested as potential surrogate markers of collagen homeostasis. To date, however, they have not been validated as markers of cartilage destruction that could be used in clinical practice.

Proteoglycans are large, negatively charged macromolecules comprising a polypeptide core with glycosaminoglycan side-chains. The largest family of proteoglycans in articular cartilage is the aggrecans, which contain abundant chondroitin sulphate and keratan sulphate side-chains. They are complexed with hyaluronic acid and so-called link protein. Their main function relates to their anionic and water-trapping properties, which provide deformability and compressibility. The ratio of collagen to aggrecan is high in the superficial layers of articular cartilage and falls progressively towards subchondral bone. Thus the surface layers have high tensile strength and resilience whereas the lower layers have higher deformability and compressibility. During load-bearing, water and solutes are squeezed out of aggrecan, which increases the relative proteoglycan concentration, providing an osmotic drive to rehydration once the load is removed.

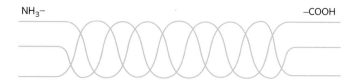

NH$_3$–   –COOH

Figure 1.2 The collagen triple helix.

Breakdown of collagen and the surrounding matrix is mediated by enzymes such as collagenase, gelatinase, stromelysin and aggrecanase, which are zinc-dependent metalloproteinases. In turn, these enzymes are controlled by tissue inhibitors of metalloproteinases (TIMPs). Thus, tissue homeostasis is maintained by carefully balanced synthetic and catabolic pathways. Cartilage thinning and breakdown (chondrolysis) can be precipitated by either excessive loading or disuse. In disease states such as RA, pro-inflammatory cytokines such as interleukin-1 (IL-1) and tumour necrosis factor-alpha (TNF-α) reduce synthesis and increase catabolism of articular cartilage, leading to rapid breakdown. In contrast, growth factors such as transforming growth factor-beta (TGF-β) and insulin-like growth factor-1 (IGF-1) stimulate synthesis of cartilage components. It is possible to measure aggrecan breakdown products in synovial fluid and blood, and these have been studied as surrogate markers of joint proteoglycan breakdown but, as with collagen markers, are not yet validated for use in the clinical setting.

Subchondral bone

The basal layer of articular cartilage is calcified and is attached directly to subchondral bone, whose structure is similar. Collagen I comprises most of the collagen present in bone, however, and is calcified with hydroxyapatite. This provides bone with both tensile and compressive strength. The remaining bone matrix is made up of proteoglycans, glycoproteins, glycosaminoglycans such as hyaluronic acid, and proteins such as osteocalcin; as in articular cartilage, these are incorporated into macromolecular complexes. Glycoproteins such as osteopontin, osteonectin and bone sialoproteins function as anchoring molecules, bridging matrix constituents such as collagen to bone cells. Bone also contains important growth factors such as IGF-1 and 2, and the bone morphogenetic proteins (BMPs) which are members of the TGF-β superfamily.

Formation and destruction. Bone contains two major cell types: osteoblasts and osteoclasts. Mesenchymal osteoblasts are critical for the synthesis of collagen and bone matrix (osteoid). Conversely osteoclasts, multinucleate cells of macrophage lineage, break down bone via a combination of lysosomal enzymes and low pH. Bone is constantly remodelled to fulfil two major functions.

- To optimize load-bearing capacity, bone is remodelled according to compressive forces acting upon it.
- Bone remodelling plays an important role in metabolic homeostasis, particularly of calcium and magnesium.

Therefore, in addition to mechanical forces, stimuli to bone formation and breakdown include circulating hormones and vitamins such as parathyroid hormone, thyroid hormone, vitamin D, calcitonin and sex hormones (Figure 1.3).

In young adults, bone formation and destruction are carefully balanced to maintain overall bone mass. In the elderly, however, and particularly in postmenopausal women, breakdown may exceed synthesis, leading to osteoporosis. Resorption is also accelerated by drugs such as corticosteroids, and by inflammation. Bone density measurements using dual emission x-ray absorptiometry (DEXA),

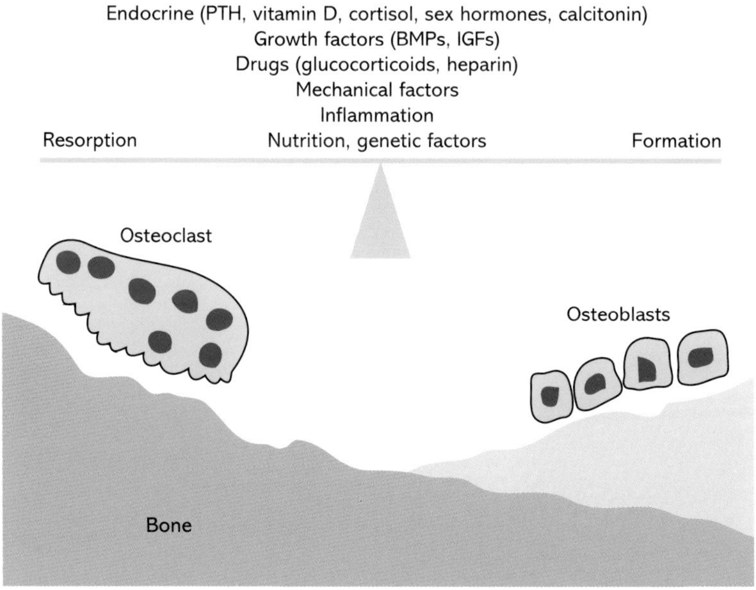

Endocrine (PTH, vitamin D, cortisol, sex hormones, calcitonin)
Growth factors (BMPs, IGFs)
Drugs (glucocorticoids, heparin)
Mechanical factors
Inflammation

| Resorption | Nutrition, genetic factors | Formation |

Osteoclast

Osteoblasts

Bone

Figure 1.3 The balance between bone synthesis and breakdown represents the integration of several influences. BMP, bone morphogenetic protein; IGF, insulin-like growth factor; PTH, parathyroid hormone.

ultrasound or quantitative computed tomography provide surrogate measures of bone strength and fracture risk. As dynamic measures, circulating bone alkaline phosphatase and osteocalcin approximate osteoblastic activity, and urinary collagen cross-links reflect collagen breakdown (from bone or cartilage), although such measurements are used predominantly as research tools at present.

Key points

- The joint is a complex organ composed of a number of specialized tissues.
- Dysregulation within any one of the tissues within the joint may precipitate specific pathologies such as osteoarthritis or osteoporosis. In RA, the primary pathological target is the synovial membrane.

Further reading

Klippel J, Dieppe P. *Rheumatology*. St Louis: Mosby-Year Book, 1998.

Maddison PJ, Isenberg D, Woo P. *Oxford Textbook of Rheumatology*. Oxford: Oxford University Press, 1998.

Ruddy S, Harris ED, Sledge CB. *Kelly's Textbook of Rheumatology*. Philadelphia: WB Saunders, 2001.

As with many common diseases, RA represents a balance between nature and nurture, in which environmental factors act upon a genetically predisposed host. It is well recognized that RA 'runs in families'. To date, however, few of the genetic and none of the environmental factors have been definitively identified.

Genetic factors

Family studies and twin studies indicate that there is a genetic susceptibility to RA, which appears to be higher in families with more severe disease. The overall genetic contribution to the aetiology is relatively small, however, at around 30%. Furthermore, unlike classical Mendelian diseases such as cystic fibrosis or sickle cell disease, RA is a polygenic and genetically heterogeneous disease. Thus, a number of different genes predispose to RA, and these may differ from patient to patient (Figure 2.1). Essentially, various combinations of polymorphisms in a selection of different genes (genotype) may predispose to the clinical picture (phenotype) that is recognized as RA. Additionally, some genes will influence severity rather than occurrence of RA. Given this complexity, and the relative importance of environmental triggers, it is hardly surprising that few genes have been consistently associated with RA.

The major histocompatibility complex (MHC) is the only genetic region that has been consistently linked to RA. This is a large genetic region on the short arm of chromosome 6 and encompasses a variety of genes (Figure 2.2). A large part of the MHC comprises the human leukocyte antigen (HLA) genes. These encode an individual's tissue type and are divided into class I (HLA-A, HLA-B, HLA-C) and class II (HLA-DR, HLA-DQ, HLA-DP) genes. The encoded proteins are critical in determining the manner in which an individual's immune system recognizes and responds to provocative stimuli, and the MHC also contains many other genes related to immune function. The strongest

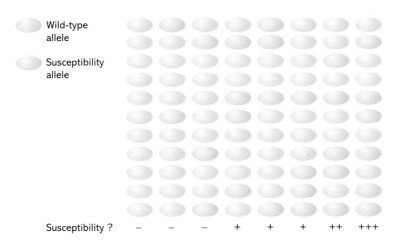

Figure 2.1 Genetics of a complex disease such as RA. Each vertical line represents an individual, for whom ten potential susceptibility genes are indicated (there are likely to be more than this). Each gene possesses a 'wild-type' (green) and a 'susceptibility' allele. For the current argument, a predisposition to RA requires the inheritance of four or more susceptibility alleles. Only one allele is shown for each gene, and it is assumed that the alternative allele is wild-type in every case. Some individuals inherit none or fewer than four susceptibility alleles and are not prone to develop RA. Others inherit four or more, resulting in a variable predisposition. Note that predisposition can involve completely different groups of genes, accounting for the phenotypic heterogeneity of RA.

link to RA within the MHC is the class II HLA region and, in particular, HLA-DRB1. HLA-DR molecules comprise an invariant alpha chain (encoded by HLA-DRA) and a highly polymorphic beta chain (encoded by HLA-DRB1), and constitute a platform upon which antigenic peptides are presented to and seen by the immune system. Particular HLA-DRB1 molecules are more common in individuals with RA, and these share a sequence in a part of the molecule that influences the peptides that are bound and therefore viewed by the immune system (Figure 2.3). This core amino acid sequence is termed the 'shared epitope'. The shared epitope probably influences the severity of RA rather than the incidence (a disease-modifying rather than a susceptibility factor) but studies are not consistent on this point.

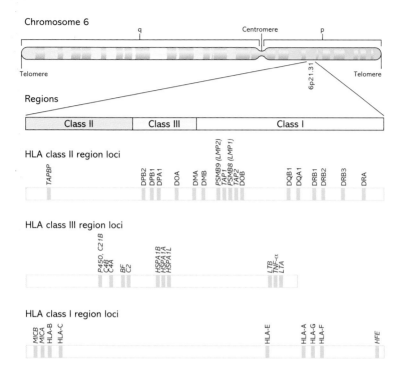

Figure 2.2 The human major histocompatibility complex (MHC) genetic locus.

Individuals that inherit two shared-epitope-containing HLA-DR molecules, however, suffer particularly aggressive disease.

It has been hypothesized that the shared epitope specifically binds a joint-derived peptide with high affinity, thereby predisposing to an autoimmune arthritis. Although the autoantigen in RA has not been definitively identified a number have been proposed (see Chapter 3) and, in most cases, specific peptides derived from these proteins can bind to HLA-DR molecules containing the shared epitope.

There are other potential explanations for this genetic association, however. For example, HLA type also biases the repertoire of T-cells generated in the thymus, and the shared epitope could, by chance, select T-cells with a particular affinity for joint antigens. The shared epitope itself could also become an autoantigen. Certain viruses and bacteria contain an identical peptide sequence within one of their proteins. An

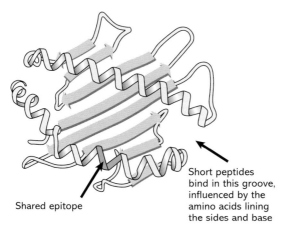

Shared epitope

Short peptides bind in this groove, influenced by the amino acids lining the sides and base

Figure 2.3

A human leukocyte antigen (HLA) DR molecule, with the approximate location of the shared epitope indicated.

immune response against the microbe could then trigger an autoimmune response against HLA-DR-expressing cells, a process termed 'molecular mimicry'.

Other genes. No other genetic locus has consistently been associated with RA, but there is some evidence implicating other genes associated with immune responsiveness. These include the gene encoding TNF-α, which is also within the MHC, particular immunoglobulin genes, and the immunoglobulin-binding Fc-γ receptors. Genetic associations with other cytokine loci, including the IL-1 gene cluster, IL-3, IL-4 and IL-10 have also been reported. Recently, a genetic locus encompassing the corticotrophin-releasing hormone (CRH) gene has been implicated in RA. The protein product of this gene plays an important role in the hypothalamo–pituitary–adrenal (HPA) axis, which is important in the stress response (see Chapter 3), but may also serve a local inflammatory role within the joint.

Infectious triggers

Although it is clear that environmental factors must trigger RA in susceptible individuals, none has been definitively identified. The most obvious candidates are infectious agents, many of which are associated with arthritic illness in both humans and in animals. For example, parvovirus B19 causes a transient illness with features of

RA in man; and Lyme disease, a chronic infection by a tick-transmitted spirochaete, has chronic joint manifestations. Lentiviruses can cause arthritis in mammals, and HIV may precipitate an arthritic illness in man. Reactive arthritis provides an obvious example of self-limiting arthritis triggered by a variety of bacterial infections; in animals, adjuvant arthritis is triggered by immunization with extracts of *Mycobacteria*.

Despite these examples, no consistent association has been found between RA and any infectious agent, and the disease does not occur in clusters or demonstrate seasonal variation. Thus, any infectious trigger may be ubiquitous in different populations, and have a high infectivity. Epstein–Barr virus (EBV) has been implicated in some studies, and certain EBV proteins provide shared-epitope-binding peptides. *Proteus mirabilis* infection has also been implicated, because of a high prevalence of serum antibodies in RA patients. *M. tuberculosis* is another potential candidate, although culture evidence is lacking. Of course, the absence of an infectious agent in arthritic tissue doesn't exclude a potential aetiological role, because a transient infection could trigger a chronic inflammatory process. For example, heat shock proteins (hsps) are a family of stress response proteins whose structures have been highly conserved through evolution. *M. tuberculosis* hsp65 is highly homologous to the human form, and an immune response against the former could trigger an autoimmune response against the latter. This is another example of molecular mimicry, and certain hsps have been implicated as autoantigens in some RA studies. It is also possible that RA is the consequence of a chronic infection with an as-yet unidentified organism.

Hormonal factors

RA is more common in women than in men, suggesting an effect of sex hormones on susceptibility. Furthermore, RA generally improves during pregnancy and may flare in the puerperium, and the age-specific incidence equalizes after the female menopause. Additionally, a number of epidemiological studies have reported a fall in the incidence of RA in women over the past 20–30 years. While the evidence is only suggestive, this has been attributed to an increase in the use of the oral contraceptive pill. No consistent effects of hormonal replacement therapy have been documented, however.

Stress and trauma have been reported to trigger RA in some individuals, which may be related to defects in HPA axis regulation (Chapter 3). This may also be consistent with genetic studies reporting linkage between RA and the CRH locus (see page 16).

Diet

Many patients report that certain foods seem to trigger episodes of arthritis. There is little consistency between patients, however, and controlled trials of dietary intervention have failed to implicate particular classes of foodstuff. These would only provide positive results, however, if patients shared a common dietary trigger whereas individuals generally identify different triggers. Starvation improves RA symptoms, and a few studies have incriminated a high-protein diet as an arthritogenic trigger. Others have reported omega–3 polyunsaturated fatty acids, as found in fish oils, to be potentially therapeutic, possibly via an effect on prostaglandin synthesis. Evening primrose oil could have similar anti-inflammatory effects, but consistent data are lacking for any of these dietary interventions.

Smoking

Smoking has been highlighted primarily as a severity factor in RA (Chapter 7), although a few studies have also implicated smoking as a RA risk factor.

A unifying model

The heterogeneity of RA may underlie the inconsistency of aetiological studies, with causation varying between patients. It is possible to construct a simple unifying model, however, based upon the known facts (Figure 2.4). In brief, a susceptible individual inherits a collection of predisposing genetic mutations. These may, for example, delay the resolution of acute inflammation and interfere with the regulation of an immune response. Any of a variety of triggers (trauma, infection, diet, smoking) could then provoke a prolonged episode of inflammation, affecting the joint or other organ systems. The relevance

Key points

- Genetic and environmental factors both play a role in the aetiology of RA but, apart from the MHC, few have been definitively associated with the disease.
- Even the MHC genetic association is uncertain, because it may be a susceptibility or a severity factor.
- The inconsistency of aetiological studies probably reflects the heterogeneity of RA as well as the influence of stochastic events; this has important implications for epidemiological studies.

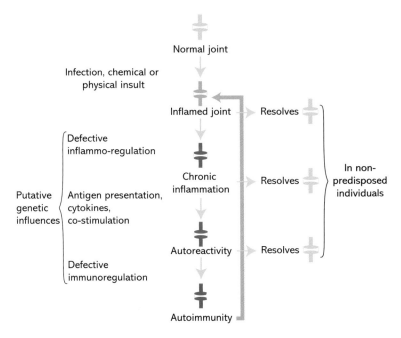

Figure 2.4 A unifying model of RA aetiology. Genetic influences on inflammatory and immune responses convert a short-lived inflammatory stimulus first into a chronic inflammatory process, and progressively into an autoreactive and autoimmune process. Note that, under normal circumstances, even autoreactivity is reversible by immunoregulatory mechanisms. Once autoimmunity is established, however, a vicious circle is maintained (blue arrow). Stochastic factors also impact on this sequence of events.

of HLA may reside in its putative ability to trigger joint autoreactivity, ultimately transforming an episode of subacute inflammation into a vicious circle of autoimmunity and chronic inflammation. In this model, different HLA types may predispose to autoimmunity in other organs, and it is common to find, for example, autoimmune thyroid disease or insulin-dependent diabetes mellitus in relatives of RA patients.

Stochastic factors. Identical twins (who inherit identical genetic material and usually share the same environment) may nonetheless be discordant for RA. This suggests that random, or stochastic, events may also be required for disease expression, further complicating aetiological studies. Possibilities include somatic genetic events such as T-cell receptor rearrangements, or epigenetic events such as x-chromosome inactivation. Additionally, immune recognition is a complex, multistage biochemical process, and it seems likely that the outcome (immune response versus no immune response) is influenced by unpredictable random events such as minor fluctuations in, for example, cell surface receptor density within the individual's 'normal range'. These concepts are difficult to prove and outside the scope of this text. Nonetheless they should probably be incorporated into models designed to explain the aetiology of diseases such as RA.

Key references

See page 30.

The fundamental pathology in RA is destruction of articular cartilage and subchondral bone by ectopic and hyperplastic synovium. A variety of models have been proposed to account for this outcome, each with some experimental support.

The synovium

The synovial membrane in RA becomes hyperplastic and, on direct visualization, may be thrown into villous-like folds (Figure 3.1). Both the lining layer and the sublining demonstrate characteristic changes in histology (Figure 3.2). In the lining layer there is an increased number of both type A and type B synoviocytes, and the intima increases from the normal 2–3 cell layers up to 10 cell layers in thickness. The sublining becomes infiltrated with immune and inflammatory cells, particularly macrophages, B- and T-lymphocytes, plasma cells and dendritic cells. Follicles of lymphoid cells may be present, resembling germinal centres of lymph nodes (Figure 3.3). Neovascularization is dramatic and an essential feature of the hyperplastic sublining layer.

As the disease progresses, the nature of the synovium changes. The synoviocytes ignore their normal tissue boundaries and migrate onto the articular cartilage, where the secretion of cytokines, and cartilage- and bone-degrading enzymes, results in the characteristic destructive

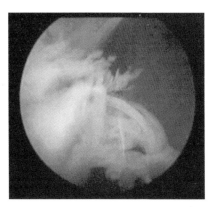

Figure 3.1 Macroscopic appearance of RA synovium on arthroscopy. The joint space is filled with hyperplastic villi and fronds of synovium. Image courtesy of Dr D Veale.

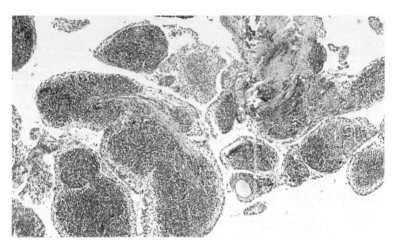

Figure 3.2 The microscopic appearance of RA synovium. The normally thin and delicate synovial membrane is invaded by inflammatory cells. There is abundant neovascularization and areas of tissue oedema. Image courtesy of Dr D Veale.

changes of RA. The invading synovium is termed pannus, and the zone of invasion is called the cartilage–pannus junction. Similar changes to these occur in the synovium lining tendons and bursae, and several of the deformities characteristic of RA result from the weakening and rupture of tendons by inflamed synovium.

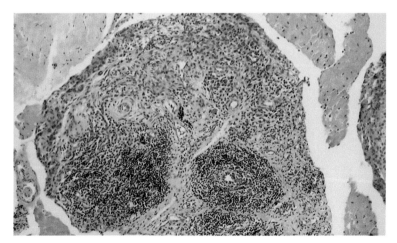

Figure 3.3 RA synovium. Nuclei are stained blue, and two clusters of lymphocytes (lymphoid follicles) are clearly shown.

Inflammatory mediators. Increased levels of cytokines are present in the RA synovium. Prominent among these are TNF-α and IL-1, but many other pro-inflammatory cytokines, including IL-6, IL-12, IL-15 and IL-18, are also present. Despite T-cell infiltration into the synovium, the overall spectrum of cytokines present is more consistent with a macrophage than with a T-cell source. When the low level of T-cell cytokines is quantified, however, there is a dominance of T helper type 1 (Th1) cytokines such as interferon-gamma (IFN-γ) relative to Th2 cytokines such as IL-4. The RA joint also contains anti-inflammatory cytokines, such as IL-10, IL-13 and TGF-β, and high levels of cytokine-neutralizing factors, such as soluble TNF-α receptors and IL-1 receptor antagonist (IL-1ra). These data suggest that a cytokine imbalance in favour of pro-inflammatory mediators may be a central pathogenic mechanism in RA (Figure 3.4). A search for pivotal regulatory cytokines showed that synovial TNF-α could influence the expression of other pro-inflammatory mediators such as IL-1 and granulocyte–macrophage colony-stimulating factor (GM-CSF). Subsequent studies in animal models and then in humans have shown TNF-α blockade to be a useful therapeutic strategy for RA (see Chapter 9). Despite its central role in the RA cytokine cascade, however, TNF-α production may be driven by T-cells. Thus, recent evidence implicates cell-to-cell contact between activated T-cells and synovial monocytes as

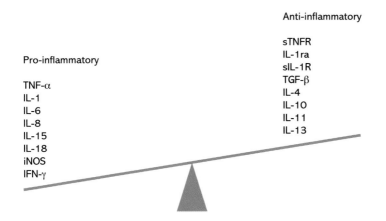

Figure 3.4 The cytokine imbalance in RA.

a stimulus to TNF-α production. Other pro-inflammatory factors present within the RA synovium include the pleiotropic mediator nitric oxide, prostaglandins and leukotrienes, and reactive oxygen intermediates. The accumulation of the last has been attributed to a form of reperfusion injury within the chronically inflamed joint secondary to elevated intra-articular pressure.

There are a number of stimuli to the prominent neovascularization of rheumatoid synovitis. These include hypoxia but, ultimately, soluble factors such as vascular endothelial growth factor (VEGF) and soluble vascular cell adhesion molecule-1 (VCAM-1) stimulate endothelial cell growth.

A number of other adhesion molecules are abundant on the vascular endothelium, including E-selectin and intercellular adhesion molecules (ICAMs). Their expression is stimulated by pro-inflammatory cytokines, such as IL-1 and TNF-α, and results in the recruitment of inflammatory cells via counter-receptors such as the integrins leukocyte function associated molecule-1 (LFA-1) and very late activation antigen-4 (VLA-4). Further progress of inflammatory cells into the joint is stimulated by chemokines, such as monocyte chemotactic protein-1 (MCP-1), IL-8 and RANTES (regulated upon activation, normal T-cell expressed and secreted; now termed MCP-2), which are highly expressed in RA synovium. These low-molecular-weight peptides provide activating and chemotactic stimuli for inflammatory cells (Figure 3.5).

Apoptosis. Physiological tissue hyperplasia, and lymphocyte proliferation during immune responses, is normally counteracted by programmed cell death, or apoptosis, preventing an overaccumulation of cells. Relatively few apoptotic cells are present in rheumatoid synovium, however, despite pro-apoptotic stimuli such as hypoxia and TNF-α. That apoptosis is actively inhibited is substantiated by the abundance of anti-apoptotic molecules, such as sentrin in synovial lining cells and Bcl-x_L in synovial lymphocytes. The survival factors have not been identified with certainty, although fibroblast-derived IFN-β is important in preventing T-cell apoptosis. Impaired synoviocyte apoptosis may result from mutation of protective oncogenes, such as

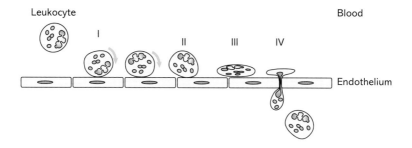

Figure 3.5 The stages of leukocyte migration into an inflammatory site. (I) Rolling along activated endothelium, mediated by selectin–selectin-ligand interactions. (II) Slowing and activation of leukocytes, mediated by endothelially located chemokines and by integrin–ligand interactions. (III) Tethering and flattening of leukocytes, mediated by integrin–ligand interactions. (IV) Transmigration of leukocytes, along a chemokine gradient and guided by integrin–connective-tissue ligand interactions.

p53, possibly secondary to the hypoxic intra-articular environment, and is central to the synoviocyte model of RA pathogenesis (see page 29).

Cartilage and bone destruction

The precise mechanism of bone and cartilage destruction in RA has not been elucidated, but a variety of destructive enzymes are secreted by pannus. Prominent among these are the various matrix metalloproteinases (MMPs) – which include collagenases, stromelysins and gelatinases – and serine and cysteine proteases, such as cathepsins. These enzymes act upon collagen and the proteoglycan matrix, thereby destroying the central structure of articular cartilage. As with the cytokines, these enzymes are controlled by physiological inhibitors such as TIMPs, again raising the possibility of a critical imbalance in RA synovium.

Other destructive factors include the cytokines TNF-α and IL-1, which activate osteoclasts to resorb subchondral bone. A further important mediator is the recently described osteoclast differentiation factor (ODF) (also referred to as TNF-related activation-induced cytokine [TRANCE], receptor activator of nuclear factor κB ligand

25

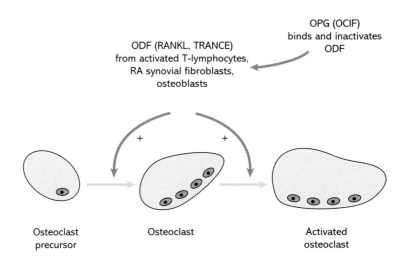

Figure 3.6 The role of osteoprotegerin and its ligands in bone resorption. OCIF, osteoclastogenesis inhibitory factor; ODF, osteoclast differentiation factor; OPG, osteoprotegerin; RANKL, receptor activator of nuclear factor κB ligand; TRANCE, TNF-related activation-induced cytokine.

[RANKL], or osteoprotegerin ligand) (Figure 3.6). This is a transmembrane protein expressed on osteoblasts and stromal cells, and a soluble form is secreted by activated T-cells. Through an interaction with membrane RANK on osteoclast precursors, ODF results in their differentiation and activation, resulting in bone destruction. Via this pathway, activated T-cells influence bone breakdown, and the combination of TNF-α, IL-1 and ODF is likely to contribute to both the peri-articular and systemic osteoporosis characteristic of RA. There is also a soluble form of RANK termed osteoprotegerin or osteoclastogenesis inhibitory factor (OCIF) which acts as a decoy receptor, protecting osteoclasts from the actions of ODF. A recombinant form of this molecule may therefore have therapeutic potential in the inhibition of bone breakdown in RA and other diseases.

Extra-articular disease in RA

Less is understood about the pathogenesis of extra-articular RA, such as rheumatoid nodules, and inflammation of the pericardium, pleura and lung parenchyma (Chapter 5). None of these sites contains synovial tissue. Histology of rheumatoid nodules reveals pallisading macrophages surrounding a necrotic core, and scattered peripheral lymphocytes. Rheumatoid factors (RhF; see pages 48–51) and, in particular, small immune complexes composed of IgG RhF dimers, have been invoked to explain the extra-articular manifestations of RA. This hypothesis suggests that IgG RhFs, produced by plasma cells within the joint, self-associate head-to-tail (Figure 3.7) and diffuse into the circulation and subsequently into the tissues. There they activate macrophages expressing Fc-γ receptors (receptors for IgG), which then produce pro-inflammatory cytokines and chemokines, leading to further inflammatory cell influx. This hypothesis is consistent with the occurrence of many RA extra-articular features at sites containing Fc-γ receptor-expressing macrophages, and has been the stimulus to ongoing trials of anti-B-cell therapy.

Rheumatoid vasculitis usually occurs in association with high levels of circulating IgM rheumatoid factor, which is highly effective at activating complement. Deposition of IgM rheumatoid factor-containing immune complexes within the perivascular tissues may therefore lead to inflammation and hence vasculitis. The presence of

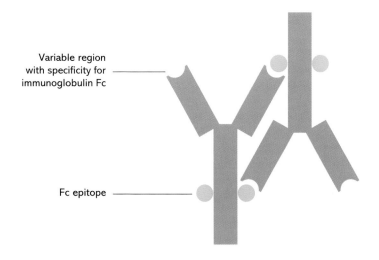

Variable region with specificity for immunoglobulin Fc

Fc epitope

Figure 3.7 The self-association of rheumatoid factors.

cryoglobulins (rheumatoid factors which precipitate at low temperatures) may lead to severe Raynaud's phenomenon and even necrosis and gangrene of the peripheries.

Neurological involvement and the hypothalamo–pituitary–adrenal axis

The symmetry of RA is highly suggestive of a neurological component to the disease, and RA synovium contains high levels of particular neuropeptides such as substance P. Their involvement in the disease process remains uncertain, but is reinforced by observations including the sparing of paralysed limbs in patients with neurological disorders such as strokes.

There is also evidence to support abnormalities in both the hypothalamo–pituitary–adrenal (HPA) and hypothalamo–pituitary–gonadal (HPG) axes in RA, including a suppressed response to stressful stimuli. Intrinsic HPA defects can also be demonstrated in some RA patients in response to conventional pharmacological stimuli, and a potential genetic linkage to the corticotrophin-releasing hormone locus has recently been described (see page 16).

Models of RA pathogenesis

A number of competing models attempt to consolidate the foregoing features. The autoimmune model views RA as a classic T-cell-mediated autoimmune disease, precipitated by autoreactivity against a joint component. Putative autoantigens include: type II collagen, a component of articular cartilage; gp39, a protein present in collagen and in monocytes; and a B-cell-derived protein called BiP (Ig heavy-chain-binding protein), which is an endoplasmic reticulum chaperonin. Due to evolutionary conservation of their structure from microbes to man, heat shock proteins have also been proposed as potential autoantigens (see page 17). Factors providing support to the autoimmune model are: the genetic link to HLA; synovial infiltration by immune cells; synovial and circulating rheumatoid factors; and efficacy of immunosuppressive drugs such as ciclosporin and leflunomide. The B-cell model of extra-articular disease (see above) also suggests an autoimmune aetiology, but invokes a primary B-cell defect.

Key points

- RA is a disease initially localized to the joint lining.
- Dominant features are synovial inflammation, and proliferation and outgrowth of the synovial lining layer, with dissolution of articular cartilage and bone.
- Pro-inflammatory cytokines are believed to play a pivotal role in pathology.
- A primary pathogenic event may reside within the immune system or the synovial lining, but none has yet been identified, and the precise pathogenesis may vary between patients.

A competing theory states that RA is primarily caused by fibroblastic synoviocytes. These cells are present in pannus and secrete many destructive factors. Furthermore, RA synovial fibroblasts exhibit characteristics reminiscent of malignant cells, such as upregulation of oncogenes, and the ability for prolonged growth with reduced contact inhibition *in vitro*. Thus, an intrinsic defect of these cells could explain many of the pathological features of RA, with chronic inflammation as a secondary phenomenon.

Lastly, macrophages are abundant in synovium taken during the earliest stages of RA. They secrete TNF-α and IL-1, two of the pivotal cytokines in RA, and studies have shown a correlation between the number of synovial macrophages and the degree of joint destruction. Thus, an intrinsic defect of these cells could underlie RA pathogenesis, although they are most readily implicated as essential players in the other models.

Key references

Feldmann M, Brennan FM, Maini RN. Role of cytokines in rheumatoid arthritis. *Annu Rev Immunol* 1996;14:397–440.

Feldmann M, Maini RN. Anti-TNF alpha therapy of rheumatoid arthritis: what have we learned? *Annu Rev Immunol* 2001;19:163–96.

Firestein G, Panayi G, Wollheim F. Rheumatoid Arthritis: *Frontiers in Pathogenesis and Treatment*. Oxford: Oxford University Press, 2000.

Fox DA. The role of T cells in the immunopathogenesis of rheumatoid arthritis – New perspectives. *Arthritis Rheum* 1997;40:598–609.

Gravallese EM, Goldring SR. Cellular mechanisms and the role of cytokines in bone erosions in rheumatoid arthritis. *Arthritis Rheum* 2000;43:2143–51.

Gregersen PK. Genetics of rheumatoid arthritis: confronting complexity. *Arthritis Res* 1999;1:37–44.

Liao HX, Haynes BF. Role of adhesion molecules in the pathogenesis of rheumatoid arthritis. *Rheum Dis Clin N Am* 1995;21:715–40.

Panayi GS, Corrigall VM, Pitzalis C. Pathogenesis of rheumatoid arthritis – The role of T cells and other beasts. *Rheum Dis Clin N Am* 2001;27:317–34.

Szekanecz Z, Koch AE. Chemokines and angiogenesis. *Curr Opin Rheumatol* 2001;13:202–8.

Tak PP, Bresnihan B. The pathogenesis and prevention of joint damage in rheumatoid arthritis - Advances from synovial biopsy and tissue analysis. *Arthritis Rheum* 2000;43:2619–33.

Yamanishi Y, Firestein GS. Pathogenesis of rheumatoid arthritis: The role of synoviocytes. *Rheum Dis Clin N Am* 2001;27:355–71.

Zhang ZX, Bridges SL. Pathogenesis of rheumatoid arthritis – Role of B lymphocytes. *Rheum Dis Clin N Am* 2001;27: 335–53.

RA is the commonest form of inflammatory arthritis. It is a heterogeneous disease and there are no pathognomonic clinical or laboratory features. It is therefore critical, when evaluating epidemiological surveys, to note the diagnostic criteria used.

Incidence and prevalence

By definition RA can start at any age from 16 upwards, although a similar disease also occurs in children (juvenile idiopathic or juvenile rheumatoid arthritis). The overall prevalence of RA in adults is around 1% in most populations, is 2–3 times higher in women and increases with age. The peak age of onset varies between studies but is probably in the fifth decade of life. RA occurs in all societies, with no clear geographical or climatic influence. On the other hand there is variation between communities. For example there is a high prevalence (approximately 5%) in some Native American populations such as the Pima Indians. Similarly, low prevalences have been reported in certain rural Chinese and Japanese communities. In Africa, a lower prevalence was reported in a rural than in an urban community. This could reflect a genuine difference in prevalence but could also be explained by other factors, such as a lower mortality from RA-associated infections in the town-dwellers or differences in the age structure of the two communities. The incidence of RA varies by as much as ten-fold between studies, and lies between 30 and 300 per 100,000 population per year. There is a suggestion that the incidence is declining, particularly in women, which some have linked to an unproven protective effect of the oral contraceptive pill.

Mortality

Traditionally, RA has been considered a chronic, disabling disease that does not shorten lifespan. This is untrue, however, and life expectancy in severe RA is reduced, on average, by 7 years for males and 4 years for females (Figure 4.1). The causes of death are largely those prevalent in society as a whole, such as atherosclerotic vascular disease, infections and malignancies. There is some evidence for accelerated atherosclerosis, which may reflect a number of factors. The reduced exercise capacity of patients with severe RA and the metabolic changes induced by corticosteroids increase predisposition. Recently, however, it has also become apparent that atherosclerosis itself has an inflammatory pathogenesis, and may therefore share predisposing factors with RA. A further argument is that subclinical vasculitis is common in RA, and that this may predispose to atherosclerosis.

The overall malignancy risk in RA is similar to that in the general population, although there is a slight increase in immune system neoplasms such as lymphomas and multiple myeloma. Along with increased mortality from infections, this reflects a degree of immune compromise, which is in part secondary to immunosuppressive drug therapy and chronic ill health. There is evidence for suppressed immunity even in early disease, however, suggesting that unidentified intrinsic disease factors also contribute. The excess mortality risk in RA is limited to patients with severe disease, usually with extra-articular manifestations.

Some recent studies have suggested that early intervention with anti-rheumatic drugs such as methotrexate has reduced the overall severity of RA, with a concomitant reduction in mortality. Methodological differences between historical and recent studies may explain this apparent improvement, however, which therefore remains contentious.

Economic impact

The costs of an illness are categorized as direct, indirect and intangible. Direct costs are the costs of medicines, and primary and secondary care. For RA, these include the costs of inpatient care, either for rehabilitation or for complications of the disease and joint surgery. Indirect costs represent the consequences of unemployment and reduced productivity. Intangible costs reflect the psychosocial consequences of RA that impact on psychological wellbeing and quality of life. The overall costs of RA have been estimated as up to $14 billion/year in the USA and £1.3 billion/year in the UK, of which only 20–25% are direct

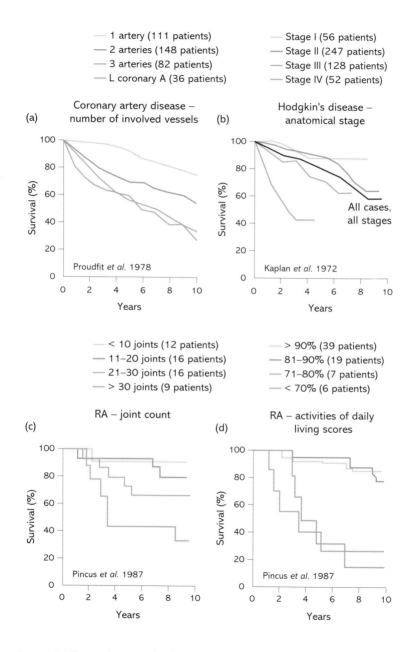

Figure 4.1 Severe rheumatoid arthritis is associated with increased mortality.
Adapted from Pincus T et al. 1994.

Key points

- RA is a global disease, present in all populations studied.
- It should not be viewed as a benign, chronic disease of the elderly. The peak age of onset encompasses the working population, and there is an associated mortality and very significant morbidity.
- The disease inflicts huge economic costs on both the individual and society.

---

costs. Of these, approximately 50% are inpatient costs, of which about 70% can be apportioned to surgery.

Work disability in RA varies between studies, but functional disability invariably occurs during the first year of disease. The initiation of therapy provides some improvement but there is then an inexorable deterioration. A recent UK-based study of patients with disease of an average duration of 6 months reported only 33% of patients with normal function at presentation, and 10% of patients with severe disability. By 5 years, 40% had normal function, but 16% had severe disability. Of those initially in paid employment, 27% were work-disabled by 5 years. Notably, 17% had already undergone orthopaedic surgery by this time. Although some studies suggest a less grim outcome, with functional stabilization following initial improvement, the above data are quite typical. By 10 years most studies report work disability rates of 40–60%.

The cost–benefit equation. Several of the newer therapies for RA have been expensive to develop and are costly to manufacture; consequently, their price can exceed $10 000/patient/year. Furthermore, some require intravenous administration, which entails additional costs. If efficacy is high, however, the need for other therapies and surgery should be reduced. If, in addition, function and employment are retained, total direct and indirect costs will be significantly reduced. Thus, the cost–benefit equation for novel RA interventions is complicated and cannot be fully ascertained for several years after their introduction into clinical practice. A corollary is the importance of adequate documentation of outcomes in patients receiving such treatments, particularly indicators of function, quality of life, and handicap (Chapter 7). Such data may be critical in the ultimate acceptance of innovative but expensive interventions of any type in a cost-conscious and resource-finite healthcare system.

Key references

Barrett EM, Scott DGI, Wiles NJ et al. The impact of rheumatoid arthritis on employment status in the early years of disease: a UK community-based study. Rheumatology 2000;39:1403–9.

Callahan LF. The burden of rheumatoid arthritis: facts and figures. J Rheumatol 1998; 25(Suppl 53):8–12.

Gabriel SE. The epidemiology of rheumatoid arthritis. Rheum Dis Clin N Am 2001;27:269–81.

Harrison B, Symmons D. Early inflammatory polyarthritis: results from the Norfolk Arthritis Register with a review of the literature. II. Outcome at three years. Rheumatology 2000;39:939–49.

Pincus T, Brooks RH, Callahan LF. Prediction of long-term mortality in patients with rheumatoid arthritis according to simple questionnaire and joint count measures. Ann Intern Med 1994;120:26–34.

Pincus T, Callahan LF, Sale WG et al. Severe functional declines, work disability, and increased mortality in 75 rheumatoid arthritis patients studied over 9 years. Arthritis Rheum 1984;27:864–72.

Sokka T, Pincus T. Markers for work disability in rheumatoid arthritis. J Rheumatol 2001;28:1718–22.

Symmons D, Harrison B. Early inflammatory polyarthritis: results from the Norfolk Arthritis Register with a review of the literature. I. Risk factors for the development of inflammatory polyarthritis and rheumatoid arthritis. Rheumatology 2000;39:835–43.

Young A, Dixey J, Cox N et al. How does functional disability in early rheumatoid arthritis (RA) affect patients and their lives? Results of 5 years of follow-up in 732 patients from the Early RA Study (ERAS). Rheumatology 2000;39:603–11.

The pathological and aetiological heterogeneity of RA is also reflected clinically, and in the earliest stages RA may be difficult to diagnose with certainty.

Early rheumatoid arthritis

No pathognomonic clinical or laboratory features of RA have been identified, and there are a number of potential differential diagnoses (Table 5.1). The diagnosis of RA rests on the presence of a constellation of clinical and laboratory features, as exemplified by the 1987 American College of Rheumatology (ACR) revised criteria (Table 5.2). A patient must fulfil at least four of these criteria. Since radiological changes and subcutaneous nodules are unusual at presentation, and approximately one-third of patients are negative for rheumatoid factor, a common presentation is a symmetrical arthritis involving the hands and wrists, associated with morning joint stiffness of at least 1 hour. Early-morning joint stiffness reflects the accumulation of inflammatory fluid in the affected joints, which recedes with an easing of symptoms as the day progresses. The symptom complex needs to be present for at least 6 weeks for the diagnosis to be made. It is important to appreciate that the ACR criteria were designed as classification criteria for patients with established disease and are less sensitive and specific in early RA. Some rheumatologists prefer to use a diagnostic tree (Figure 5.1), which may be more sensitive but less specific. The commonest joints to be affected by RA at presentation are the metacarpo-phalangeal (MCP) and proximal interphalangeal joints of the hands, and the metatarso-phalangeal (MTP) joints of the feet. This distribution of joint involvement results in early functional impairment and slowed mobility, to which excessive fatigue and malaise may contribute. Objectively there is swelling of affected joints, which may be accentuated by inflammation of overlying tendon sheaths, particularly in the hands. Range of joint motion is restricted by synovitis of both the joints themselves and the tendon sheaths.

TABLE 5.1

Differential diagnosis of recent-onset polyarthritis or polyarthralgia

Inflammatory synovitis

- Rheumatoid arthritis
- Psoriatic arthritis
- Enteropathic arthritis
- Reactive arthritis
- Reiter's syndrome
- Ankylosing spondylitis
- Post-viral arthritis
- Inflammatory osteoarthritis
- Polyarticular gout
- Pseudogout
- Connective tissue disease (e.g. systemic lupus erythematosus, systemic sclerosis)
- Vasculitis (e.g. Wegener's granulomatosis, Henoch–Schönlein purpura)
- Sarcoidosis
- Behçet's disease

Non-inflammatory conditions

- Generalized osteoarthritis
- Fibromyalgia

Metabolic

- Osteomalacia
- Hyperparathyroidism
- Renal bone disease (in chronic renal impairment)
- Hypothyroidism

Chronic infection

- Subacute bacterial endocarditis
- Hepatitis B
- Human immunodeficiency virus

Miscellaneous

- Paraneoplastic
- Multiple myeloma
- Polymyalgia rheumatica
- Septic arthritis (not usually polyarticular)

While this is the commonest presentation of RA, there are many other possibilities. The disease can affect any synovial joint, and larger joints such as the elbows, shoulders or knees may also be involved. Unusual symptoms reflect the involvement of joints such as the crico-arytenoid joint of the larynx, with resultant hoarseness. Inflammation of synovium at extra-articular sites leads to tenosynovitis and bursitis.

TABLE 5.2

1987 American College of Rheumatology diagnostic criteria for rheumatoid arthritis

Four of the following seven criteria must be met, and criteria 1–4 must have been present for at least 6 weeks:

1. Morning stiffness in and around joints lasting 1 hour or more before maximal improvement

2. Soft tissue swelling (arthritis) of three or more joint areas

3. Swelling (arthritis) of the proximal interphalangeal, metacarpo-phalangeal, or wrist joints

4. Symmetrical arthritis

5. Subcutaneous nodules

6. Positive test for rheumatoid factor

7. Radiographic erosions and/or periarticular osteopenia in hand and/or wrist joints

Source: Arnett FC et al. 1988

Tenosynovitis further compounds functional impairment, particularly of the hands and wrists. Bursitis causes pain at juxta-articular sites: for example at the hip, where trochanteric bursitis is common. The tempo of onset is also variable, ranging from an acute, dramatic presentation in up to a third of cases to a more classical insidious clinical picture, which may have been present for several months before the patient seeks medical advice. Fatigue and malaise may be prominent features and in some cases may overshadow the articular symptoms.

The course of early disease is also variable, ranging from progressive, unremitting symptoms spreading to additional joints to less common 'palindromic' symptoms which may last from just hours to days before remitting, only to reappear at a later date. In the elderly, prominent myalgia may add to diagnostic confusion and some individuals present with symptoms indistinguishable from polymyalgia rheumatica before progressing to more typical RA. In such patients, the coexistence of myalgic and arthritic symptoms further compounds disability.

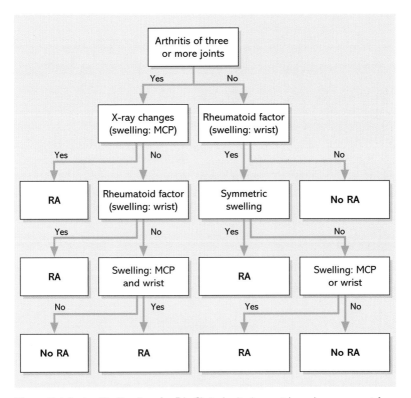

Figure 5.1 A classification tree for RA. Clinical criteria must have been present for at least 6 weeks and observed by a physician. Surrogate variables that can be used when the alternative is not available are given in parentheses. MCP, metacarpo-phalangeal joints.

Established rheumatoid arthritis

The picture of established RA is changing as a result of effective therapies being used earlier in the disease. Thus, the signs may be similar to those of early disease, although more joints generally become affected as the disease becomes established. The hallmarks of established RA, however, are the characteristic deformities that result from a combination of synovitis and resultant joint damage, tenosynovitis and ligamentous laxity (Figure 5.2).

Hands. In the hands the swan-neck, boutonnière and z thumb deformities each represent tendon slippage with an altered axis of traction that compromises joint motion. Subluxation and ulnar

39

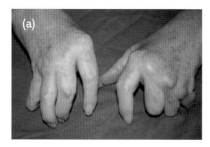

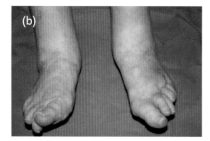

Figure 5.2 Characteristic appearance of the hands and feet in RA. The hands demonstrate subluxation and ulnar deviation at the metacarpo-phalangeal joints, flexion deformities of the fingers, and rheumatoid nodules over pressure points. The feet show swelling and valgus deformities at the ankles, flattening of the medial longitudinal arches, clawing of the toes, and scars from previous surgery.

deviation at the MCP joints, and subluxation at the wrist are also characteristic features of established RA. Flexor tenosynovitis is additionally associated with 'triggering' of the fingers.

Feet. In the feet, the subtalar joint and talo-navicular joint are more commonly affected than the ankle joint itself. A valgus deformity at the subtalar joint results in flattening of the longitudinal arch and pes planus. Disease of the MTP joints and associated tendons results in splaying and clawing of the toes followed by subluxation. Consequent pressure on the metatarsal heads during walking results in the characteristic symptom of 'walking on pebbles'. When examining the feet, inspection of the plantar surface may reveal calluses at unusual sites that, in turn, suggest impaired foot mechanics.

Neuromuscular complications. In established RA, there is significant muscle wasting around affected joints. In the upper limbs, this may be prominent in the hands and forearms, compounded by cervical spine disease and associated radiculopathy or by compression neuropathies.

RA can affect the cervical spine at any level, leading to various sequelae. The best known, although not the commonest, is atlanto-axial subluxation. This arises from synovitis affecting the articulation between the odontoid peg of the axis and the transverse ligament of the atlas. The design of this articulation enables rotatory movement but, with disruption of the transverse ligament, anterior–posterior movement also becomes possible with the danger of spinal cord compression by the odontoid peg during neck flexion (Figure 5.3). The peg may also separate from the axis completely and migrate cranially towards the foramen magnum, causing basilar invagination and compression of the cervical cord and medulla.

More commonly, synovitis of the apophyseal joints at lower cervical levels leads to subluxation and spinal cord compression. The resultant myelopathy is characterized by upper-limb symptoms and signs in a radicular distribution, alongside 'long tract' pyramidal and sensory features affecting the lower limbs. In some cases, cervical spine disease is relatively asymptomatic until the sudden appearance of neurological deficits. A high index of suspicion is therefore necessary, and surveillance radiology should be considered in patients with evidence of cervical spine RA, with a view to stabilization surgery for progressive subluxation at any level. The cervical spine is also vulnerable in RA patients undergoing laryngeal intubation as part of a general anaesthetic, or requiring upper gastrointestinal endoscopy, and a full assessment is mandatory in such cases.

Entrapment neuropathies are also common causes of pain, neurological symptoms and muscle wasting in RA. By far the

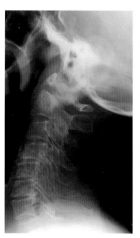
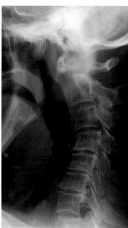

Figure 5.3 Atlanto-axial subluxation. Anterior subluxation of the atlas on the axis becomes obvious during neck flexion (right), which is likely to compromise the spinal canal. Images courtesy of Dr P Robinson.

41

commonest is carpal tunnel syndrome due to median nerve compression by synovitis at the wrist, which may even be a presenting feature. Similarly, synovitis at the elbow can cause entrapment of the ulnar nerve or the posterior interosseous branch of the radial nerve, the latter causing wrist drop. Again, these features can severely compromise already-reduced hand function. At the ankle, entrapment of the medial peroneal nerve in the tarsal tunnel may cause pain or numbness of the medial border of the foot (tarsal tunnel syndrome).

In patients with rheumatoid vasculitis, involvement of the vasa nervorum may present as a glove-and-stocking sensorimotor neuropathy.

Extra-articular features

Extra-articular features of RA usually occur in rheumatoid factor positive individuals with severe, active joint disease. Occasionally, however, serious extra-articular involvement or even vasculitis arises in patients whose arthritis appears to have remitted or 'burnt out'. In particular, corneal 'melts' (see page 45) frequently arise in elderly patients with minimal inflammatory joint symptoms. There is no obvious explanation for this dichotomy, which emphasizes the importance of regular and systematic review of RA patients by a specialist throughout the course of their disease.

Systemic features. The commonest extra-articular manifestation is the rheumatoid nodule. These are usually subcutaneous and occur most commonly overlying pressure points. They are firm and non-tender unless infected, and range in size from a few millimetres in diameter to several centimetres (Figure 5.4). Common sites for nodules are the extensor surface of the forearms and over pressure points of the wrists, hands (Figure 5.2a) and feet. Nodules may also occur at non-cutaneous sites. In the lungs a solitary nodule may mimic a malignant tumour. In contrast, massive and multiple nodules may be seen in ex-coal miners with pneumoconiosis (Caplan's syndrome). When localized to the sclera of the eye, nodules may cause thinning and, rarely, perforation of the globe (scleromalacia perforans). Nodules often improve with effective treatment of RA, but methotrexate may worsen nodulosis in some patients despite improvement in articular disease activity.

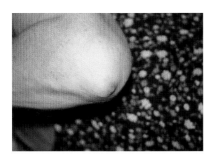

Figure 5.4 A rheumatoid nodule at the elbow. A small rheumatoid nodule has ulcerated. Additional subcutaneous nodules are evident on the extensor surface of the proximal forearm.

Lymphadenopathy is also associated with active RA and may coexist with systemic features such as fever and weight loss, raising the possibility of lymphoma. Histology, however, generally reveals 'reactive changes' of mild follicular hyperplasia.

Abnormal liver function tests (LFTs) are also a frequent finding in active RA, with mild and non-specific changes on liver biopsy. It is important to distinguish disease-related changes in LFTs from abnormalities induced by therapies.

Amyloidosis, secondary to the deposition of serum amyloid A protein (an acute-phase reactant) in the tissues, is now a rare complication of RA, and reflects prolonged, active disease. It can present with multi-organ symptoms and signs, involving the kidney, intestines, liver, spleen and heart. Carpal tunnel syndrome is a more benign presentation.

Haematological complications. Active RA is often associated with anaemia. This is usually normochromic and normocytic and a consequence of chronic inflammation. Iron deficiency may coexist, however, secondary to drug-induced gastrointestinal blood loss. Other causes of anaemia in RA include an autoimmune haemolytic anaemia, which is uncommon, and drug-induced marrow suppression. In common with other inflammatory conditions, thrombocytosis may occur in active RA. In Felty's syndrome, patients with RA develop splenomegaly with features of hypersplenism (pancytopenia in the peripheral blood). Neutropenia is usually more marked than either thrombocytopenia or anaemia. This is a serious complication, associated with recurrent bacterial infections, chronic leg ulcers and increased mortality. The cause of Felty's syndrome is not understood, but some patients have an excess of natural killer (NK)-cell-like large granular lymphocytes in their peripheral blood.

Chest disease. Lung involvement is common in RA, with pleural disease being present in up to 50% of post-mortem examinations. Patients may experience pleuritic chest pain and pleural effusions, but lung involvement is often asymptomatic. An inflammatory alveolitis (interstitial pneumonitis) is less common but can lead to irreversible pulmonary fibrosis if untreated. It generally starts in the lower lobes and presents as a dry cough, or as dyspnoea on exertion. Certain anti-rheumatic drugs can also cause an inflammatory alveolitis, particularly methotrexate.

Serositis is also a common post-mortem finding in the pericardium. Again, this is frequently asymptomatic but pericardial chest pain and effusions may occur. Myocardial involvement is less common but nodules can cause a myocarditis, and varying degrees of heart block.

Ocular complications. The commonest ocular complication is keratoconjunctivitis sicca, or dry eyes (xerophthalmia). This is usually a consequence of secondary Sjögren's syndrome, and may be associated with dry mouth (xerostomia) and vaginal dryness, the latter possibly leading to dyspareunia. The diagnosis is supported by a positive Schirmer's test, in which an absorbent paper wick is placed just inside the lower eyelid to measure tear production. In Sjögren's syndrome less than 5 mm of the wick becomes wet in 5 minutes. In patients with coexistent xerostomia, histology of a lip salivary gland biopsy reveals a lymphocytic infiltrate destroying the glandular tissue.

The episclera lies between the sclera and the conjunctiva, and inflammation (episcleritis) presents with redness and irritation of the eye. Clinically there is a nodular or diffuse brownish-red 'blushing' of the episcleral blood vessels. The condition is benign and usually self-limiting. More sinister is the occurrence of scleritis, which is easily distinguishable as an intensely painful inflammation of the sclera itself. Again this can be diffuse or nodular but, in contrast to episcleritis, necrosis and thinning of the sclera may occur, ultimately leading to perforation of the globe. In scleromalacia perforans, on the other hand (see page 42), thinning is often painless and only presents when the blue-black pigment epithelium becomes visible through the affected translucent sclera. Occasionally the sclera perforates, with protrusion of the pigment epithelium.

Similar processes affecting the cornea result in keratitis which may be acutely painful (acute necrotizing keratitis). A more insidious and less inflammatory process occurs at the periphery of the cornea (peripheral ulcerative keratitis) resulting in the condition known as 'corneal melt' (Figure 5.5). Destructive processes affecting the sclera and cornea are ophthalmological emergencies, and RA patients should receive regular ophthalmological screening, particularly if they have xerophthalmia, which predisposes to melting.

The skin. Raynaud's symptoms are common in the general population but have an increased prevalence in patients with RA and other connective tissue diseases. The diagnosis requires a triphasic colour change during cold exposure. The extremities turn intially white, then blue and ultimately pink due to reactive hyperaemia. Occasionally the

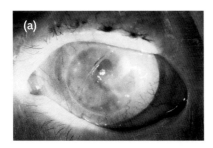

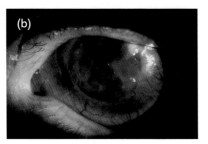

Figure 5.5 Corneal melt. (a) There is thinning of the lateral aspect of the left cornea, with a surrounding inflammatory infiltrate. (b) The area of ulceration is highlighted by the use of fluorescein eye drops. Images courtesy of Mr A Morrell.

> **Key points**
>
> - RA has a variety of articular and extra-articular manifestations.
> - Its spectrum ranges from mild, easily controlled disease to progressive, destructive disease with life- and organ-threatening extra-articular complications.
> - Patients require close and regular monitoring by a specialist clinician.

severity of the condition results in digital ulceration and must then be differentiated from cryoglobulinaemia or rheumatoid vasculitis.

Rheumatoid vasculitis most commonly affects the small arteries, particularly in the hands and feet, leading to nail-fold infarcts of the fingers and toes (Figure 5.6). Leg ulcers may also be vasculitic in RA (Figure 5.7). More sinister is the involvement of medium-sized arteries, leading to digital gangrene. At this stage multi-organ involvement is possible, including the mesenteric, coronary or cerebral vessels, although renal involvement is rare.

Osteoporosis is a common and often underdiagnosed complication of RA. From disease onset, bone mass decreases for multiple reasons, such as increased bone resorption (see Chapter 3), immobility and

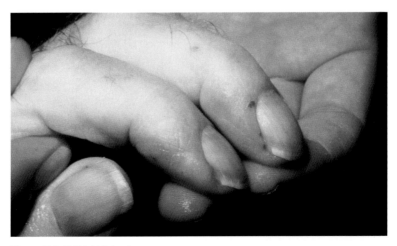

Figure 5.6 Nail-fold infarcts.

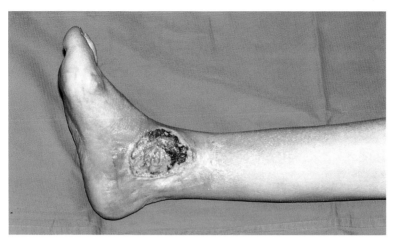

Figure 5.7 A vasculitic leg ulcer in a patient with RA. The ulcer has punched-out edges and a necrotic base.

glucocorticoid therapy. There are currently few guidelines for the management of low bone mass in RA, but it is important to be aware of risk factors, such as glucocorticoid therapy, and to treat accordingly. In RA, a combination of osteopenia and impaired gait is a recipe for fractures secondary to falls, with a further reduction in mobility and function.

Key references

Arnett FC, Edworthy SM, Bloch DA *et al*. The American Rheumatism Association 1987 revised criteria for the classification of rheumatoid arthritis. *Arthritis Rheum* 1988;31:315–24.

Kim JM, Weisman MH. When does rheumatoid arthritis begin and why do we need to know? *Arthritis Rheum* 2000;43:473–84.

Saraux A, Berthelot JM, Chales G *et al*. Ability of the American College of Rheumatology 1987 Criteria to predict rheumatoid arthritis in patients with early arthritis and classification of these patients two years later. *Arthritis Rheum* 2001;44:2485–91.

Although there are no pathognomonic clinical or laboratory features of RA, certain investigations, such as a positive rheumatoid factor (RhF) or characteristic x-ray changes, support a clinical diagnosis. It is possible, however, to establish a diagnosis of RA in the presence of entirely normal investigations. Initial investigations (Table 6.1) are guided, on the one hand, by the differential diagnosis (see Table 5.1 on page 37) and, on the other, by predictors of damage or prognosis (see Chapter 7).

Immunological investigations

RhF is an autoantibody with specificity for the Fc portion of normal immunoglobulin (IgG) (Figure 3.7). IgM RhF is present in 75–80% of RA patients during the course of their disease, although it may be absent at presentation. In contrast, its presence may predate the onset of RA by several years. Its precise role in the pathogenesis of RA is unclear, but it is associated with more aggressive disease and extra-articular manifestations. RhF is not specific for RA, but may accompany other autoimmune diseases, various acute and chronic infections and certain malignancies (Table 6.2). The serum titre of RhF does not correlate with disease activity, except in patients with vasculitis, who tend to have a high titre (Chapter 3). Conventional tests for RhF measure immunoglobulin of IgM isotype, however, whereas models of RA pathogenesis implicate IgG or IgA RhF. These isotypes may therefore be more informative but are difficult to measure and not routinely available. They do seem to be better predictors of a poor long-term prognosis (Chapter 7) than IgM RhF. Occasionally, a RhF is present in serum that precipitates at low temperatures. This is detectable as a cryoglobulin and may be associated with vasculitis and severe Raynaud's phenomenon.

Other autoantibodies may also be present in patients with RA. Although not routinely measured at present, antibodies to certain citrullinated peptides such as filaggrin, a basic protein of the stratum

TABLE 6.1

Investigation of recent-onset polyarthritis or polyarthralgia

(Investigations in parentheses are dictated by the clinical picture)

Inflammatory markers

- C-reactive protein
- Plasma viscosity
- Erythrocyte sedimentation rate

Haematology

- Full blood count with differential white cell count

Biochemistry

- Renal function, including urine analysis
- Hepatic function
- Calcium, phosphate
- Uric acid
- (Thyroid function tests)
- (Serum angiotensin-converting enzyme)
- (Vitamin D, parathyroid hormone)
- (Creatine kinase)

Immunology

- Rheumatoid factor
- Anti-nuclear factor
- Serum immunoglobulins, including electrophoresis
- (Anti-neutrophil cytoplasmic antibody)
- (Complement)
- (Cryoglobulins)
- (Tissue typing - HLA-DR, HLA-B27)

Virology/microbiology (when clinical picture dictates)

- Parvovirus serology
- Rubella serology
- Influenza serology
- *Mycoplasma* serology
- Antistreptolysin-O titre
- Hepatitis B serology
- HIV serology
- *Yersinia* serology
- *Campylobacter* serology
- Stool/urethral cultures

Synovial fluid

- To exclude infection
- Positively or negatively birefringent crystals

End-organ investigation

- Radiology of appropriate joints
- (Chest x-ray)
- (Electrocardiogram)
- (Echocardiogram)
- (Pulmonary function tests)
- (Nerve conduction studies/electromyography)
- (Dual x-ray absorptiometry scan)
- etc.

TABLE 6.2

Associations of a positive rheumatoid factor

Infection

- Acute infection, e.g. infectious mononucleosis
- Chronic bacterial infection, e.g. subacute bacterial endocarditis, tuberculosis, leprosy
- Parasitic infections, e.g. malaria, schistosomiasis
- Vaccination

Inflammatory disease

- Rheumatoid arthritis
- Connective tissue diseases, e.g. systemic lupus erythematosus, Sjögren's syndrome
- Cryptogenic fibrosing alveolitis
- Chronic active hepatitis
- Cryoglobulinaemia

Malignancy

- Lymphoma
- Leukaemia
- Myeloma
- Solid tumours

Health

- A positive rheumatoid factor at low titre is common in the healthy population

corneum, are present in 40–50% of RA patients and are more specific but less sensitive than RhF. These include the so-called anti-keratin antibodies and anti-perinuclear factor, and may be useful diagnostically in patients who are RhF negative. Anti-nuclear antibodies are present in approximately 40% of RA patients, usually at low titre, and have minimal diagnostic or prognostic value. Anti-neutrophil cytoplasmic antibodies (ANCA, usually p-ANCA with specificity for lactoferrin), have been reported in up to 50% of RA patients in some studies. A potential association with more aggressive disease or vasculitis requires confirmation.

Radiology

X-rays are often normal in RA at presentation, or may just show soft-tissue swelling and periarticular osteoporosis around affected joints. Subsequently, classical juxta-articular erosions provide more robust diagnostic information (Figure 6.1). In later disease, erosions spread to the subchondral areas, joint-space narrowing occurs and ultimately subluxation, secondary osteoarthritis and even bony ankylosis may ensue. The rate of development of these changes varies greatly between patients and depends both on therapy and also on the aggressiveness of the underlying disease. Earliest changes are usually seen in the hands or feet, and x-rays of the hands, wrist and feet are usually performed at presentation. If changes are present these are important prognostically

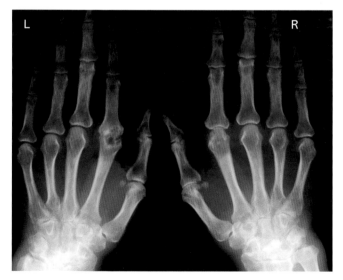

Figure 6.1 Radiological damage secondary to RA. The bones are osteopenic, and there is a large erosion of the left second metacarpo-phalangeal joint. There is loss of joint space and definition throughout the carpal bones and at the radiocarpal joints bilaterally. Image courtesy of Dr P Robinson.

51

(Chapter 7) but may also help in the differential diagnosis from, for example, inflammatory osteoarthritis, psoriatic arthritis and gout.

In contrast to conventional x-rays, modern imaging modalities may show significant abnormalities in the patient with a very recent onset of joint symptoms. These include magnetic resonance imaging (MRI) and high-resolution ultrasound (HRUS), although at present both modalities are at the stage of validation. MRI detects the water content of tissues, and readily demonstrates articular and peri-articular structures (Figure 6.2). Additionally, MRI can capture structural information in several planes, and computer-generated 3-dimensional reconstructions are possible. In the patient with early RA, inflamed synovium appears as a high signal on T2-weighted images, and enhances further with the paramagnetic contrast agent gadolinium-DTPA. Furthermore, bone marrow oedema adjacent to the joint surface appears to presage erosion development.

A major disadvantage of MRI is the cost of the equipment and individual scans. It is also a relatively lengthy procedure, requiring the patient to lie still for a considerable period of time in a semi-enclosed space. This may be physically difficult, and some patients also find the procedure claustrophobic. Newer magnet designs are addressing some

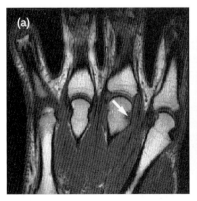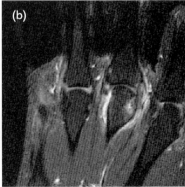

Figure 6.2 Coronal MR image of the metacarpo-phalangeal joints in early RA. The left panel is a T1-weighted image, which illustrates a bony erosion (arrow). Corresponding bone oedema, as well as adjacent synovial inflammation, is shown on a T2-weighted fat-suppressed image (right panel). Image courtesy of Dr P Conaghan.

of these issues, but the procedure remains largely a research tool at present. In contrast, MRI is the investigation of choice for imaging the rheumatoid cervical spine, where it provides high-resolution images of the spinal canal and cord. Similarly, osteonecrosis (avascular necrosis) is readily diagnosed using MRI, for example at the hip. This may occur as a complication of the disease process or be secondary to therapy with corticosteroids.

In Europe, although not in the USA, HRUS is becoming a popular rheumatological imaging technology. It is a relatively inexpensive investigation following initial investments in equipment and training. Like conventional ultrasound, HRUS depends on the relative absorption and reflection of ultrasonic waves by adjacent tissues. In early RA, it is possible to detect small joint effusions and subclinical synovitis. In addition, bone cortical defects are detectable in patients without x-ray erosions (Figure 6.3). HRUS is also useful for imaging tendons and soft tissues, for example at the shoulder or ankle where symptoms may be secondary to arthritis, bursitis, tendinitis or fasciitis. Furthermore, ultrasound can be used to guide the placement of injections. This improves accuracy compared with that of conventional 'blind' injections (for example into the shoulder), and also permits injections into joints that lack reliable bony landmarks, such as the hip. In Europe, rheumatologists themselves are becoming trained in the use of HRUS, which may become a clinic room or bedside aid to the diagnosis, assessment and management of joint disease.

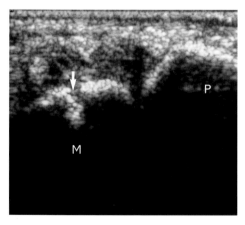

Figure 6.3 Longitudinal ultrasound image through a metacarpo-phalangeal joint of a patient with RA. There is a cortical break (arrow) on the metacarpal head (M) consistent with an erosion. P, proximal phalanx. Image courtesy of Dr R Wakefield.

Key points

- There are no pathognomonic tests for RA, and investigations may be completely normal at presentation.
- In the acute setting the investigation of polyarthritis is guided primarily by the differential diagnosis.
- Conventional x-rays may provide diagnostic information but are less sensitive than MRI and HRUS; these last two, however, remain research tools at present.
- In the chronic setting, investigations are useful for determining disease activity, monitoring therapy, and documenting joint damage.

Synovial fluid

Synovial fluid examination is not helpful for the diagnosis of RA. Joint aspiration and microbiological examination is imperative, however, if superadded infection is suspected. This is not uncommon, particularly in the patient taking immunosuppressive drugs, and requires prompt diagnosis and treatment. Infection presents as disproportionate inflammation in one or more joints, with or without systemic symptoms, and the patient may feel that a distinct process is present in the affected joint. Gout or pseudogout are alternative possibilities, also diagnosed by synovial fluid examination. It is important to appreciate that the macroscopic appearance of synovial fluid is not a reliable guide to the underlying diagnosis. Fluid from acutely inflamed joints secondary to gout or pseudogout may be thick and purulent, whereas fluid from an infected RA joint may appear only slightly cloudy. The definitive diagnosis of these conditions requires Gram stain, crystal analysis using polarized light, and culture of the synovial fluid.

Monitoring RA

In established RA, investigations are aimed at determining disease activity, documenting damage, and monitoring drug therapy. A normochromic, normocytic anaemia suggests poorly-controlled disease, as does a low serum albumin. There is no indication to repeat RhF titres in a seropositive patient, because they do not correlate with disease activity (see above), but a seronegative patient may convert to seropositivity during the course of their illness. Any patient with poorly controlled disease, particularly if taking glucocorticoid therapy, should be considered for osteoporosis screening by DEXA or an alternative. It is reasonable to repeat radiology of the hands, wrists and feet every 2 years to document stabilization or progression of erosive disease. Other radiological investigations should be guided by the clinical picture. The assessment of ongoing RA is discussed in more detail in Chapter 7.

Key references

See pages 12 and 64.

When a patient develops RA, they are keen to understand their long-term outlook. RA can result in severe disability and a dependent existence. Mild disease, however, is readily controlled with relatively non-toxic drugs or may even spontaneously remit, with no permanent handicap. It is not possible to provide a completely accurate picture for each patient, but a number of prognostic factors have now been defined. It is also important to gauge accurately the current status of a patient, in order to decide on the need for, and effectiveness of, therapy, and to draw valid conclusions when new and existing therapies are compared.

Prognosis

There are two aspects of RA prognosis to consider. First, which patients with inflammatory synovitis of recent onset will develop chronic and progressive, as opposed to mild and self-limiting, disease? Second, of the former group, which factors predict more severe joint damage? With regard to the first question, recent studies suggest that inflammation of the MCP joints lasting for longer than 12 weeks is the simplest predictor of chronicity, and symptoms that resolve before this time tend not to recur. At present there is no laboratory marker that can provide equivalent information at an earlier time point.

Factors which are associated with more severe damage are listed in Table 7.1. These include simple demographic factors such as female sex, an older age at disease onset, or a lower formal educational level, each of which imparts a worse prognosis. Smoking has also been associated with more erosive disease. At presentation, a longer duration of symptoms, functional limitation (see below), or a raised acute-phase response are all associated with a worse prognosis. Adverse immunogenetic features include seropositivity for RhF (Chapter 6), a tissue type that includes HLA genes encoding the 'shared epitope' (Chapter 2), or a reduced capacity to oxidize sulphur (sulphoxidation

TABLE 7.1

Poor-prognostic factors in rheumatoid arthritis

- Female sex
- Older age at disease onset
- Longer disease duration at presentation
- Low formal educational level
- Smoker
- Poor functional status at presentation
- Raised acute-phase response at presentation
- Positive rheumatoid factor status
- Shared-epitope-positive HLA type
- Reduced ability to oxidize sulphur (poor sulphoxidation status)
- X-ray-evident joint damage at presentation

status). Autoantibodies against citrullinated peptides have also been linked with a worse prognosis (Chapter 6), but this requires confirmatory studies. Lastly the presence of x-ray erosions at presentation is, not surprisingly, a poor prognostic sign.

Patients that are seen in academic referral centres are likely to have more severe disease and usually possess more of the above-mentioned poor-prognostic factors. On the other hand certain subtypes of RA, such as polymyalgic onset at an advanced age, appear to have a more favourable prognosis.

Assessment of ongoing RA

The assessment of RA is objective and subjective. For example, a swollen-joint count and an acute-phase response provide useful objective measures. On the other hand, entirely subjective features such as fatiguability, or the duration of early-morning joint stiffness, may be more important from the patient's perspective. Additionally, satisfaction with medical management may depend more upon the patient's functional capabilities. These will encompass personal (washing, dressing, preparing a meal), social (e.g. ability to leave the house and attend a party), and economic (ability to remain in their current occupation in a full-time capacity) activities. Importantly, the same physical impairment can result in varying degrees of disability. Thus, a deformity affecting the non-dominant hand will be of more consequence to a musician than to a writer. Furthermore, the same deformity in an elderly person may prevent them from dressing themselves and be socially isolating. Psychological factors including coping strategies and illness perception are also important determinants of disability, as are social perspectives. Thus, the elderly person living alone will be more disabled than if they have a partner to help them dress. Anxiety and depression also have major impacts on the degree of disability experienced.

Assessing function. Functional impairment may be evident at presentation. At this stage of the disease it usually reflects the degree of joint inflammation, although later the cumulative effects of damage to tendons, ligaments, cartilage and bone also contribute. A number of self-completion questionnaires that focus on function have been designed and validated. Some are condition-specific, such as the Stanford Health Assessment Questionnaire (HAQ) or the Arthritis Impact Measurement Scale (AIMS), whereas others are generic, such as the short form 36 (SF36). These questionnaires collect information along a number of dimensions (e.g. self-care, hand function, mobility, work and play) that relate to the activities of daily living and psychosocial functioning (Figure 7.1). They are useful tools for assessing current disease status but also carry prognostic significance (see above). Some instruments, such as the modified HAQ (mHAQ), specifically seek changes in function since the previous assessment, via 'transitional' questions. Others, such as the McMaster Toronto Arthritis (MACTAR) Patient Preference Questionnaire, adopt a patient-specific perspective, and attempt to measure personal handicap. Thus, the patient nominates specific roles pertinent to their personal situation and, at each assessment, rates their ability to fulfil those roles.

A simple alternative to questionnaires is to observe and measure patients completing simple tasks such as walking a set distance, fastening and unfastening buttons, or by assessing grip strength using an inflatable cuff. Patients can also be allocated to specific

Please tick the ONE best answer for your abilities

At this moment, you are able to:	Without any difficulty	With some difficulty	With much difficulty	Unable to do
Dress yourself, including tying shoelaces and fastening buttons?				
Get in or out of bed?				
Lift a full cup or glass to your mouth?				
Walk outdoors on flat ground?				
Wash and dry your entire body?				
Bend down to pick up clothing from the floor?				
Turn normal taps on or off?				
Get in and out of a car?				

Figure 7.1 Example of a self-assessment functional questionnaire for RA patients. From: Pincus T *et al. Ann Intern Med* 1989;110:259–66.

TABLE 7.2

American College of Rheumatology functional classification of rheumatoid arthritis

Class I: Completely able to perform usual activities of daily living (self-care, vocational, and avocational)

Class II: Able to perform usual self-care and vocational activities, but limited in avocational activities

Class III: Able to perform usual self-care activities, but limited in vocational and avocational activities

Class IV: Limited in ability to perform usual self-care, vocational and avocational activities

Usual self-care includes dressing, feeding, bathing, grooming and toileting. Vocational (work, school, homemaking) and avocational (recreational and/or leisure) activities are patient-desired and age- and sex-specific.

Source: Hochberg MC *et al.* 1992

'functional classes' (Table 7.2), but these are relatively insensitive to short-term change.

Quality of life. Quality of life (QOL) encompasses a number of dimensions, including physical, social, psychological and economic aspects. Functional capabilities are an important determinant of QOL, and some questionnaires address both. Generic examples include the Nottingham Health Profile and the SF36, whereas the rheumatoid arthritis quality of life (RAQOL) instrument was designed specifically for patients with RA.

Composite scores. RA is a complex disease and cannot be assessed using a single measure. Therefore, in accordance with the variable manifestations and outcomes of RA, composite assessment criteria have been devised, although debate continues regarding the 'minimal data set' needed to provide a reliable picture of the individual patient. The Paulus criteria and, more recently, the ACR response criteria were designed for assessing outcomes in the clinical trials setting. The ACR response criteria measure changes from baseline in the number of tender and swollen joints, acute-phase response, a functional measure (e.g. HAQ score), visual analogue scale for pain, and global assessment of disease by patient and physician, also on a visual analogue scale. A 20% improvement in swollen and tender joint counts, and in three of the remaining five parameters, represents an ACR20 response. This is the minimum required for efficacy in most trials. ACR50 and ACR70 responses are calculated in a similar fashion.

While useful for monitoring clinical trials, these scores have not been validated in the routine clinical setting. Furthermore, they must relate to a particular baseline, and a given improvement may be more difficult to achieve from a less active baseline. Thus, a 20% improvement from a baseline of 5 swollen joints may be more difficult to achieve than from a baseline of 20 swollen joints.

In contrast, the disease activity score (DAS, Table 7.3) provides a continuous variable which does not require reference to a baseline.

The DAS is a complex measure that was derived by studying a number of disease activity criteria in patients with variable disease activity, and applying assorted statistical measures, including discriminant analysis and multiple regression analysis. Because of its continuous nature, a patient can be assigned a meaningful DAS at any stage of their disease, and interpatient comparisons can also be made. Some rheumatologists now record DAS routinely at each clinic visit. This provides a longitudinal quantitative measure of RA activity by which to judge the effectiveness of current management and the need for adjustment. In the clinical trial setting, improvement targets can be defined as both a reduction in DAS and also a target level of DAS, providing for good, moderate and nil improvements. The DAS28 is a modification based on 28 swollen and tender joints (Table 7.3).

Radiology. Functional impairment in chronic RA is influenced by the amount of joint damage. This can be assessed using conventional x-rays, according to a number of semiquantitative grading systems such as the Larsen and Sharp scores. In essence, these quantify radiographic change in a number of prespecified joints of the hands (and the feet in the modified Sharp score) to provide a single score. Recent modifications focus on erosions and joint-space narrowing independently, and also discriminate between new joints affected versus progression in previously affected joints. Most patients with RA

TABLE 7.3

The disease activity score (DAS) and DAS28

$$DAS = 0.53938\sqrt{(RAI)} + 0.06465(S44) + 0.330(lnESR) + 0.00722(GH)$$
$$DAS28 = 0.56\sqrt{(T28)} + 0.28\sqrt{(S28)} + 0.70(lnESR) + 0.014(GH)$$

DAS28, DAS including the 28-joint count. RAI, Ritchie Articular Index, a graded joint tenderness score based on 53 joints. S44, ungraded joint swelling based on 44 joints. lnESR, natural logarithm of erythrocyte sedimentation rate. GH, patient's assessment of general health in millimetres on a visual analogue scale of 100 mm. T28, ungraded joint tenderness count based on 28 joints. S28, ungraded joint swelling count based on 28 joints

Sources: Van der Heide *et al.* 1993; Van Gestel AM *et al.* 1998

Key points

- RA can be assessed using objective clinical scores such as swollen-joint counts, biochemical and radiological parameters such as acute-phase response and joint x-rays, and subjective measures of pain, function and handicap.
- Most information is captured in composite scores such as the DAS.
- Quality of life is of overriding importance to the patient, and should always be considered during routine assessments.

eventually develop joint damage, and the rate of progression and severity are both relevant to functional impairment.

While specific, x-ray damage occurs slowly and is an insensitive measure over the short term. Thus, although a gold standard for structural outcome, it is of limited use in early disease or for monitoring the effects of therapy in the short term. In contrast, HRUS and MRI can detect changes in synovitis and bone marrow oedema over periods of weeks to months (Chapter 6). While currently at the stage of validation, these modalities may become valuable adjuncts for the monitoring and assessment of RA.

Biochemical markers of damage. Quantifiable markers of tissue destruction should provide a complementary and dynamic adjunct to radiological monitoring as the complex biochemistry of synovium, bone and cartilage is elucidated and tissue-specific markers defined. For example, serum osteocalcin levels provide a dynamic measure of osteoblastic activity, and type I collagen c-telopeptide levels of bone resorption. Urinary deoxypyridinolone cross-links may also reflect bone damage. In contrast, no consistently useful assays are yet available for measuring proteoglycan synthesis or breakdown. A number of assays have been developed for quantifying cartilage oligomeric matrix protein (COMP) as a serum marker of cartilage damage, but these continue to be refined and validated. At present, none of the above measurements has sufficient sensitivity or specificity to be applied routinely in the clinic.

Remission

Remission is the ultimate aim of RA therapy and is defined according to strict criteria, established in 1982 by Pinals *et al.* (Table 7.4). These criteria are very exacting, however, and are unlikely to be fulfilled by patients with joint damage. Alternative criteria are being defined and debated, including the use of synovial imaging. Thus, synovitis may be present on MRI or HRUS in the absence of clinically obvious inflammation. This may underlie the progression of bony damage in some patients during apparent clinical 'remission'. When using the DAS, remission is defined as a score of less than 1.6.

TABLE 7.4

American College of Rheumatology criteria for clinical remission of rheumatoid arthritis

A minimum of five of the following for at least 2 consecutive months:

1. Morning stiffness not to exceed 15 minutes

2. No fatigue

3. No joint pain

4. No joint tenderness or pain on motion

5. No soft-tissue swelling in joints or tendon sheaths

6. Erythrocyte sedimentation rate (Westergren's method) less than 30 mm/hour (females) or 20 mm/hour (males)

Clinical remission cannot be diagnosed in the presence of manifestations of active vasculitis, pericarditis, pleuritis, myositis, and/or unexplained recent weight loss or fever

Source: Pinals RS *et al.* 1982

Key references

Combe B, Dougados M, Goupille P et al. Prognostic factors for radiographic damage in early rheumatoid arthritis, a multiparameter prospective study. *Arthritis Rheum* 2001;44:1736–43.

Emery P, Salmon M, Bradley H et al. Genetically-determined factors as predictors of radiological change in patients with early symmetrical arthritis. *BMJ* 1992;305:1387–9.

Green M, Marzo-Ortega H, McGonagle D et al. Persistence of mild early inflammatory arthritis: the importance of disease duration, rheumatoid factor, and the shared epitope. *Arthritis Rheum* 1999;42:2184–8.

Hochberg MC, Chang RW, Dwosh I et al. The American College of Rheumatology 1991 revised criteria for the classification of global functional status in rheumatoid arthritis. *Arthritis Rheum* 1992;35:498–502.

Jansen LM, den Horst-Bruinsma IE, van Schaardenburg D et al. Predictors of radiological joint damage in patients with early rheumatoid arthritis. *Ann Rheum Dis* 2001;60: 924–7.

Kaltenhauser S, Wagner U, Schuster E et al. Immunogenetic markers and seropositivity predict radiological progression in early rheumatoid arthritis independent of disease activity. *J Rheumatol* 2001;28: 735–44.

Pinals RS, Masi AF, Larsen RA et al. Preliminary criteria for clinical remission in RA. *Bull Rheum Dis* 1982;32:7–10.

Van der Heide DMFM, van't Hof M, van Riel PLCM et al. Development of a disease activity score based on judgement in clinical practice by rheumatologists. *J Rheumatol* 1993;20:579–81.

Van Gestel AM, Haagsma CJ, van Riel PLCM. Validation of rheumatoid arthritis improvement criteria that include simplified joint counts. *Arthritis Rheum* 1998;41:1845–50.

Van Gestel AM, van Prevoo MLL, van't Hof MA et al. Development and validation of the European League Against Rheumatism response criteria for rheumatoid arthritis. Comparison with the preliminary American College of Rheumatology and the World Health Organisation/ International League Against Rheumatism Criteria. *Arthritis Rheum* 1996;39:34–40.

Wolfe F, Cush JJ, O'Dell JR et al. Consensus recommendations for the assessment and treatment of rheumatoid arthritis. *J Rheumatol* 2001;28:1423–30.

The ultimate goal of RA management is to reduce pain and discomfort, prevent deformities and loss of normal joint function, and to maintain normal physical, social, and emotional function and capacity to work. Management begins with effective communication between physician and patient.

If one accepts the paradigm that both the acute and chronic consequences of RA are due to persistent, misdirected and inadequately controlled inflammation that causes tissue destruction and loss of function, then prolonged and complete control of the abnormal inflammatory process is the fundamental objective of management. Unfortunately, even with the newest therapeutic options, most patients achieve only partial suppression of inflammation and many lose therapeutic benefit after an initial good response. The management of persistent or recurrent rheumatoid inflammation and disability therefore continues to be a challenge. It remains to be determined whether the future addition of more potent specific interventions in the inflammatory process (see Chapters 9 and 10) will be able to solve this problem without disarming host defences against infections and tumours. Because the exact cause of RA remains unknown, treatment is currently directed against various components of the chronic inflammatory process, rather than the underlying aetiology.

Non-pharmacological approaches

Reduction of joint stress can be accomplished by local rest of an inflamed joint. Weight reduction, splinting, use of walking aids and specially designed utensils can all significantly reduce stress on specific joints. During significant disease flares, vigorous activity should be avoided, although full range of motion of joints should be maintained by a graded exercise programme to prevent contractures and muscular atrophy. The role of physical and occupational therapy, podiatry, nursing educational programmes, and vocational rehabilitation cannot be overemphasized. Rest, splinting of involved joints, adaptive equipment, appropriate exercise programmes, orthotics, foot care and bespoke shoes, and nutritional and physiological support are all essential ingredients of a successful treatment regimen.

Pharmacological approaches – overview

The traditional 'pyramid' approach to the treatment of RA was to begin with symptomatic treatment of inflammation using non-steroidal anti-inflammatory drugs (NSAIDs) in addition to rest and corticosteroid injections. If the disease did not significantly improve with these simple treatments, then more potent disease-modifying anti-rheumatic drugs (DMARDs) were added. Recent studies have revealed, however, that DMARD therapy early in the course of RA slows disease progression more effectively than delayed use. This has led to a general agreement that inflammation of RA should be controlled as completely as possible and as soon as possible by the early introduction of DMARDs, and that this control should be maintained for as long as possible. The currently approved drugs for treating RA are listed in Table 8.1. Most of these drugs require monitoring for the prompt detection of potential adverse effects. The precise monitoring recommendations vary from centre to centre, however. In the UK the British Society for Rheumatology provides guidelines for the commonly used drugs, but local guidelines also exist in many regions. The American College of Rheumatology has developed guidelines for the use and monitoring of RA therapies.

Non-steroidal anti-inflammatory drugs

NSAIDs are probably the most frequently prescribed drugs in the treatment of patients with RA, at least early in the disease process. The major effect of these agents is to reduce joint pain and improve joint function. There is no evidence that NSAIDs have any effect on the underlying disease process, and exacerbation of symptoms occurs quickly after metabolic elimination of the drugs. They are rarely, if ever, treatment for RA in isolation and without DMARD therapy.

The major therapeutic effect of NSAIDs relates to their ability to suppress the synthesis of prostaglandins by inhibiting the enzyme cyclooxygenase (COX). It has recently been discovered that COX exists

TABLE 8.1

Drug therapy for rheumatoid arthritis

Non-steroidal anti-inflammatory drugs (COX-non-selective and COX-2-selective)

Analgesics

Corticosteroids

- Systemic (oral or parenteral)
- Intra-articular

Disease-modifying anti-rheumatic drugs

- Methotrexate
- Antimalarials: hydroxychloroquine, chloroquine
- Sulfasalazine (sulphasalazine)
- Gold salts
- Leflunomide
- Ciclosporin (cyclosporin[e])
- D-penicillamine
- Azathioprine
- Cyclophosphamide
- Tumour necrosis factor inhibitors
  - etanercept
  - infliximab
- Interleukin-1 inhibitors
  - anakinra

COX, cyclooxygenase

in two isoforms: COX-1 and COX-2. COX-1 is expressed constitutively in many tissues and is primarily responsible for the production of prostaglandins by vascular endothelium, platelets and gastric mucosa, leading to haemostatic and cytoprotective effects. It is also important for the regulation of renal blood flow. COX-2 is undetectable in most normal tissues; its expression increases during development of inflammation, and can be induced by several pro-inflammatory stimuli.

Recently, more selective COX-2 inhibitors have been approved for use in RA or osteoarthritis. Their principal benefit is the production of analgesic and anti-inflammatory effects comparable to those of the non-selective NSAIDs, but with lower risk of serious gastrointestinal adverse reactions and without prolongation of the bleeding time. Renal side-effects may still occur, however, as a result of constitutive COX-2 expression in the kidney. In the UK, the National Institute for Clinical Excellence (NICE) has issued guidance on the use of COX-2 inhibitors (Table 8.2).

Corticosteroids

Corticosteroids have a long history in the treatment of many rheumatic diseases and they are still a key element in the management of RA. They usually produce rapid and potent suppression of inflammation, with improvement in fatigue, joint pain and swelling. A randomized, double-blind, placebo-controlled study demonstrated a decrease in

TABLE 8.2

Summary of the National Institute for Clinical Excellence (NICE) guidelines on COX-2 antagonists

COX-2 selective inhibitors should be used in preference to standard NSAIDs only in patients who may be at 'high risk' of developing serious gastrointestinal adverse effects. These include:

- those aged 65 years and older
- those using concomitant medications known to increase the likelihood of upper gastrointestinal adverse effects (e.g. corticosteroids, anticoagulants)
- those with serious comorbidity (e.g. cardiovascular disease, diabetes, hypertension, renal or hepatic impairment)
- those requiring the prolonged use of maximum recommended doses of standard NSAIDs.

The risk of NSAID-induced complications is particularly increased in patients with a previous history of gastroduodenal ulcer, gastrointestinal bleeding or gastroduodenal perforation. The use of even a COX-2 selective agent should therefore be considered especially carefully in this situation.

NSAIDs, non-steroidal anti-inflammatory drugs

progression of joint erosion in patients with early RA administered low-dose daily prednisolone (7.5 mg) for 2 years. Joint destruction resumed when prednisolone was discontinued. Prednisolone (prednisone in the USA) is most frequently used for RA at a dose of 5–10 mg once daily to minimize adrenal suppression and metabolic side-effects. The therapy is often initiated in patients with significant functional decline and active disease while awaiting the full therapeutic effect of disease-modifying anti-rheumatic drugs (DMARDs). Corticosteroids are rarely used without concomitant DMARD therapy.

Once started, corticosteroid therapy is difficult to discontinue, and tapering should be gradual to avoid disease flares: e.g. 0.5–1.0 mg/day every few weeks to months. For this reason some rheumatologists prefer to use a single parenteral dose of a depot steroid preparation (e.g. methylprednisolone acetate or triamcinolone acetonide) when rapid control of inflammation is required. This can be administered by intramuscular injection, with efficacy lasting for 6–8 weeks. Intra-articular steroid injections are particularly useful for controlling, with minimal systemic effects, a local flare in joints that show disproportionate involvement.

Side-effects. The side-effects of corticosteroids, in particular the associated immunosuppression and catabolic consequences, limit their long-term use especially in high doses. Careful surveillance and preventive interventions are needed to avoid undesired complications. Periodic assessment for steroid-induced osteoporosis has become a standard of care for patients receiving chronic corticosteroid therapy. Patients with and without additional osteoporosis risk factors should undergo regular bone densitometry to assess fracture risk. The greatest risk of bone loss occurs during the first 6–12 months of corticosteroid use. If bone densitometry is not readily available, some rheumatologists recommend prophylactic treatment, for example with a bisphosphonate, in any patient commencing prednisolone treatment and who is likely to receive a dose of 75 g or higher for at least 6 months.

Disease-modifying anti-rheumatic drugs

All patients with RA are candidates for DMARD therapy. DMARDs have in the past been reserved for patients not improving with NSAIDs, but DMARD therapy is now initiated at the time of diagnosis. DMARDs lack an analgesic effect, and it may take weeks or months before any clinical benefit is recognized. They often only moderate the disease process, and some level of chronic inflammation usually persists. The disease generally recurs after the drug is discontinued. These agents may reduce the acute-phase response and most have now been shown to slow the rate of progression of joint erosions and disability, to a variable extent.

Antimalarials (chloroquine and hydroxychloroquine) are commonly used drugs with a favourable toxicity-benefit profile. Chloroquine is more popular in mainland Europe and appears to be more potent but more toxic than hydroxychloroquine, which is used in the USA and UK. Hydroxychloroquine (200–400 mg daily) is often used in early mild disease and as background therapy when another DMARD is started. There are no data available to prove that hydroxychloroquine alone reduces or prevents radiological damage from RA.

Side-effects. The most serious potential adverse event is ocular toxicity secondary to retinal deposits, particularly with chloroquine. This is extremely rare with hydroxychloroquine, but it is recommended that patients undergo an ophthalmology examination before starting therapy and at intervals thereafter.

Methotrexate, as a result of its favourable efficacy and toxicity profile, low cost and predictable benefit, has become the most commonly used DMARD for RA in the USA. More than 50% of patients taking methotrexate continue the drug for more than 5 years, which is longer than for any other DMARD. Despite its efficacy, the precise mechanism of action of methotrexate in RA is uncertain. Because of variable enteral absorption, many rheumatologists will prescribe parenteral (subcutaneous or intramuscular) methotrexate following ineffective oral therapy and before changing to an alternative DMARD. Unfortunately, plasma level testing is not routinely available. The effective oral dose ranges from 7.5 to 25 mg once weekly. It is essential that the patient understands that dosing is weekly and not daily, as the latter will result in potentially fatal bone marrow suppression.

Contraindications and monitoring. Use of methotrexate in patients with renal insufficiency or on dialysis should be avoided. Guidelines for monitoring of patients with RA while on methotrexate have been established. Baseline tests for all patients prior to initiation of therapy should include a full blood count (FBC) (complete blood cell count, CBC, in the USA), serum creatinine and LFTs, and chest x-ray. Hepatitis B and C serologies are recommended in the USA, and some rheumatologists also perform pulmonary function testing particularly when there is a history of pre-existing pulmonary disease. Haematological monitoring and LFTs (transaminases, alkaline phosphatase) should subsequently be performed on a regular basis. Women of childbearing age must be aware that methotrexate has potential for teratogenesis and should practise effective birth control.

Side-effects. Nausea, mucositis, bone marrow suppression, and hepatocellular injury are the main side-effects. Less common complications include interstitial pneumonitis and fibrosis, and opportunistic infections may rarely occur. Gastrointestinal symptoms may be avoided by the concomitant use of folic acid or a change to parenteral administration. Folic acid may also reduce hepatic enzyme abnormalities associated with methotrexate use.

Sulfasalazine (sulphasalazine) is a conjugate of a salicylate and a sulfapyridine molecule and is a highly popular DMARD in Europe. The usual dose is 1 g twice daily. In addition to an anti-inflammatory effect due to the salicylate component, sulfasalazine appears to have immunomodulatory effects, and has an efficacy similar to that of methotrexate. It is frequently used in combination with other DMARDs.

Side-effects. Gastrointestinal symptoms are the most common side-effects, and are often resolved with dose attenuation. Haematological consequences include aplastic anaemia, agranulocytosis, or haemolytic anaemia, and monitoring of the FBC is recommended on a regular basis, in addition to LFTs.

Leflunomide is a recently approved DMARD with immunomodulatory properties. It is an isoxazole prodrug that is rapidly converted in the gastrointestinal tract to an active metabolite following oral administration. The active metabolite binds to and reversibly inhibits the enzyme dihydroorate dehydrogenase (DHODH), the rate-limiting enzyme in *de novo* pyrimidine synthesis, which is essential for lymphocyte turnover. Leflunomide therefore has inhibitory effects on lymphocyte proliferation and has demonstrated efficacy in the management of RA. The rate of progression of radiographic damage during phase III studies was comparable to that with methotrexate or sulfasalazine. It takes about 7–8 weeks for this drug to reach steady-state levels in the blood. To decrease this time, a loading dose of 100 mg/day for 3 days is recommended, followed by a maintenance dose of 10–20 mg/day.

Side-effects. Adverse events include bone marrow toxicity, reversible alopecia, skin rash, stomatitis, diarrhoea, hypertension and elevation in liver enzymes. Routine monitoring of FBC, liver function tests and blood pressure are required. Leflunomide is also teratogenic. It has an extremely long half-life and, if required, its elimination can be accelerated with cholestyramine or activated charcoal.

Gold compounds, because of their effectiveness in suppressing synovitis, were the most popular disease-modifying agents in the 1970s and early 1980s. However, due to their toxicity and the existence of many new alternatives, they are less often used today. The parenteral preparations currently in use are aurothioglucose (Solganol, available in the USA) and sodium aurothiomalate (Myocrisin), administered intramuscularly. An initial test dose of 10 mg should be administered before commencement of weekly therapy of 50 mg. The dosing interval can be increased once efficacy is established. Auranofin, an oral preparation, is less effective than intramuscular gold and rarely used. The exact mechanism of action has not been definitively established, but it is postulated that gold compounds act at many points in the sequence of inflammatory events.

Side-effects. The most common adverse effects of gold are mucocutaneous reactions, including stomatitis, pruritis, and various forms of dermatitis. Proteinuria may occur and is usually mild, although rarely reaches the nephrotic range. Leukopenia, thrombocytopenia, or aplastic anaemia are rare but potentially fatal consequences. FBC and urinalysis should be performed prior to each injection.

Penicillamine is also rarely prescribed today in hospital practice. It has a similar adverse effect profile to that of gold salts, and side-effects occur frequently. When used, it is initiated at a dose of 125–250 mg daily, with slow escalation to a maintenance dose of 500–750 mg daily if tolerated.

Ciclosporin (previously cyclosporin[e]) is a drug that inhibits T-cell function and is a mainstay in preventing rejection of transplanted organs. In RA it is effective as monotherapy and as an adjunct to methotrexate. In general, however, it is reserved for refractory cases of RA, primarily because of its nephrotoxic adverse events which preclude its widespread use.

Cytotoxic drugs, including azathioprine and cyclophosphamide, are generally reserved for patients with refractory RA who have failed conventional therapy. Despite their efficacy profile, they are little used today in RA, because of their toxicity and existence of new alternatives. Cyclophosphamide, however, is used in patients with rheumatoid vasculitis or organ-threatening extra-articular disease such as interstitial pneumonitis. The usual mode of administration is by intermittent intravenous 'pulses', often accompanied by intravenous corticosteroid.

Combination therapy. The use of DMARD combinations when a single agent fails to control clinical symptoms of RA is generally accepted by rheumatologists. The question remains whether to initiate treatment in a 'step-up' approach by adding new agents in patients in whom a single drug has failed or whether to begin with combination therapy early in the disease and use a 'step-down' method once disease is under control. Evidence from a randomized, placebo-controlled clinical trial showed promising results with increased efficacy and acceptable toxicity using the triple combination of methotrexate, sulfasalazine and hydroxychloroquine in established RA. In a further combination study, step-down prednisolone, in combination with methotrexate and sulfasalazine, was more efficacious than sulfasalazine alone in early RA, an effect that persisted for up to a year from cessation of steroids. Combinations of biological agents with methotrexate have been studied and also found to be beneficial (see Chapter 9). Further studies will determine the optimal clinical use of combination therapy.

Surgery

Remarkable progress has been made in the past twenty years in orthopaedic procedures, which have improved the quality of life of many patients. In particular, joint replacements have become the standard of care for large joints (e.g. hip, knee) with end-stage disease and complete loss of cartilage.

In general there are two types of indication for surgery. The first is to deal with irreversibly damaged tissues and specific disease complications. This category includes joint replacements but also, for example, forefoot surgery for intractable pain secondary to rheumatoid deformities. Repair of damaged tendons, for example at the shoulder, also falls under this heading, as would the removal of problematic rheumatoid nodules. The second category includes prophylactic surgery to prevent deformity and loss of function. Synovectomy, for example, is currently accepted as a treatment for refractory joint or tendon sheath involvement before the destruction of surrounding tissues ensues. This is of particular clinical relevance at the hand, where flexor tendon involvement is common. Similarly, stabilization of the cervical spine will prevent progressive myelopathy in the predisposed patient (see page 41).

The optimal timing of, and potential benefit to be gained from, orthopaedic surgery in the RA patient requires skilled judgement. Similarly, both local and systemic disease activity must be optimally controlled peri-operatively. It follows that pre- and post-operative assessment and care requires a multidisciplinary approach involving not only surgeon and rheumatologist, but also occupational therapist and physiotherapist. Most important of all, the patient must be absolutely clear as to the indication for surgery (relief of pain, preservation of

Key points

- There is no algorithm for the treatment of RA.
- NSAIDs, and corticosteroids, provide symptomatic relief but should rarely be used in isolation.
- Disease-modifying anti-rheumatic drugs (DMARDs) are now the mainstay of pharmacological therapy. These include antimalarials, methotrexate, sulfasalazine, leflunomide, gold compounds, ciclosporin and cytotoxic drugs.
- Early treatment with DMARDs is essential to avoid irreversible joint damage, and combinations may be required.
- DMARDs are generally safe with appropriate monitoring, but adverse events are potentially life-threatening if missed.
- Optimal therapy also includes access to allied health professionals such as physiotherapists, occupational therapists and podiatrists.
- The need for, and timing of, surgery requires skilled judgement.
- Consequently, the patient with RA is optimally managed from disease onset by a rheumatologist and their team.

function, or both) and likely outcome. For example, pain-relieving elbow surgery may improve quality of life but not upper limb function.

Conclusions regarding therapy

There is no algorithm for the treatment of RA. The decision about which drugs to use and when to use them remains individualized and is determined by the degree of disease activity, functional status, and the toxicity profile of a potential regimen. The patient must be fully educated about treatment options, and decisions regarding drug therapy must be by mutual agreement.

The concept of long-term therapy with NSAIDs or corticosteroids while awaiting a natural remission is no longer acceptable. Early control of the disease process is essential to minimize irreversible joint damage and functional disability. Rheumatologists today initiate DMARD therapy (with single agents or in combination) as soon as the diagnosis of RA is secure, without requiring the presence of radiographic changes. For this reason, it is critical that patients are referred for specialist assessment as soon as the diagnosis of RA is suspected, and even before the results of investigations are available.

The rheumatologist must serve as an advocate for the patient with regard to treatment and drug monitoring programmes. In the USA, this is particularly important in light of potential restrictions, due to changes in the healthcare reimbursement system and managed care. With the advent of expensive biological treatments (Chapter 9), economic considerations may also become relevant in the UK.

Patients treated by rheumatologists have a slower rate of disease progression, and less joint damage and disability, than those not receiving care from the arthritis specialist. The expertise of the rheumatologist is in advising drug regimens, referring to rehabilitation specialists, and recognizing the importance and timing of orthopaedic consultation and procedures.

Key references

Boers M, Verhoeven AC, Markusse HM et al. Randomised comparison of step-down prednisolone, methotrexate and sulphasalazine with sulphasalazine alone in early rheumatoid arthritis. Lancet 197;350:309–18.

Kirwan JR, Byron M, Dieppe P et al. The effect of glucocorticoids on joint destruction in rheumatoid arthritis. N Engl J Med 1995;333:142–6.

Lindroth Y, Brattstrom M, Bellman I et al. A problem-based education program for patients with rheumatoid arthritis: evaluation after three and twelve months. Arthritis Care Res 1997;10:325–32.

O'Dell JR, Haire CE, Erickson N et al. Treatment of rheumatoid arthritis with methotrexate alone, sulfasalazine and hydroxychloroquine, or a combination of all three medications. N Engl J Med 1996;334:1287–91.

Strand V, Cohen S, Schiff M et al. Treatment of active rheumatoid arthritis with leflunomide compared with placebo and methotrexate. Leflunomide Rheumatoid Arthritis Investigators Group. Arch Intern Med 1999;159:2542–50.

Tugwell P, Pincus T, Yocum D *et al*. Combination therapy with cyclosporine and methotrexate in severe rheumatoid arthritis. The methotrexate–cyclosporine combination study group. *N Engl J Med* 1995;333:137–41.

Weinblatt ME, Kremer JM, Coblyn JS *et al*. Pharmacokinetics, safety, and efficacy of combination treatment with methotrexate and leflunomide in patients with active rheumatoid arthritis. *Arthritis Rheum* 1999;42:1322–8.

Advances in bench research and biotechnology over the past several years have led to a better understanding of the pathogenesis of RA. Now there is a significant interest in 'biological response modifiers (BRMs)' as potential therapeutic agents for RA. BRMs are recombinant proteins that target specific molecules in the immune and/or inflammatory process. Examples include monoclonal antibodies (mAbs), recombinant cytokines and cytokine inhibitors, as well as fusion proteins consisting of biological 'targeting' segments fused with toxins or immunoglobulins (Table 9.1).

Tumour necrosis factor inhibitors

An important advance in the treatment of RA has been the targeting of TNF-α. In the last 3 years, the US Food and Drug Administration (FDA) and the European Agency for the Evaluation of Medical Products (EMEA) have both approved two TNF-α antagonists for the treatment of refractory RA: etanercept and infliximab.

The TNF-α precursor is found in a variety of cells throughout the body. Macrophages appear to be the primary site of active TNF-α production in RA, via TNF-α converting enzyme (TACE)-mediated cleavage of the precursor molecule. After being shed from the cell surface, soluble TNF-α molecules aggregate into trimolecular complexes that subsequently bind receptors on a variety of cells, including fibroblasts, leukocytes, and endothelial cells. Two TNF-α receptors have been described: the p55 (also called p60) receptor and the p75 (also called p80) receptor. TACE also cleaves the extracellular domain of the cell surface TNF receptors, forming soluble TNF receptors (sTNFRs). These circulating sTNFRs are then free to bind the trimolecular TNF complexes, rendering them biologically inactive; thus, the sTNFRs function as natural inhibitors of TNF-mediated inflammation.

A variety of physiological functions have been ascribed to TNF–TNF-receptor interactions. TNF-α blocks the action of

TABLE 9.1

Biological response modifiers studied in RA*

Agents targeted against T-cells

- Murine anti-CD4 mAb

- Humanized anti-CD4 (non-depleting) mAb

Agents targeted against T-cell activation markers

- Anti-IL-2 receptor mAb

Co-stimulatory molecule antagonists

- CTLA4-Ig

- Anti-CD40 mAb

- Anti-CD40 ligand mAb

Cytokines and cytokine antagonists

- p75 TNF-receptor-immunoglobulin fusion protein (etanercept)

- PEGylated p55 TNF receptor dimeric protein

- Chimeric anti-TNF mAb (infliximab)

- Humanized anti-TNF mAb (adalibamab)

- IL-1 receptor antagonist (anakinra)

- Soluble IL-1 receptor

- Anti-IL1 mAb

- IL-1 TRAP

- IL-1 converting enzyme inhibitor

- Anti-IL6 mAb

- Recombinant interferon beta

- Anti-IL-12 mAb

Agents targeted at signalling cascades

- MAP kinase inhibitors

Complement inhibitors

- Anti-C5a mAb

Adhesion molecule antagonists

* Currently in use or being evaluated in patients with rheumatoid arthritis.
mAb, monoclonal antibody; IL, interleukin; MHC, major histocompatibility complex;
CTLA, cytotoxic T-lymphocyte-associated protein; TNF, tumour necrosis factor;
PEG, polyethylene glycol; MAP, mitogen-activated protein; ICAM, intercellular adhesion molecule

lipoprotein lipase, causing severe cachexia in experimental models of chronic infection. Additionally, TNF-α induces programmed cell death (apoptosis) and stimulates the release of several other pro-inflammatory cytokines, including IL-6, IL-8, and IL-1. It also induces the release of matrix metalloproteinases (MMPs) from fibroblasts, chondrocytes and neutrophils, activates osteoclasts, and upregulates the expression of endothelial adhesion molecules, leading to the migration of leukocytes into extravascular tissues.

Etanercept is a genetically engineered molecule containing two human soluble p75 TNF receptors linked to the Fc portion of human IgG1 (Figure 9.1). The clinical utility of etanercept in adults with RA has been assessed in placebo-controlled, double-blind, randomized clinical trials involving over 500 patients. Etanercept produced significant improvements in all measures of disease activity including the rate of progression of joint damage. The recommended dosage for adults is 25 mg by subcutaneous injection twice weekly. Etanercept is approved for both adults and children with RA. Etanercept has been shown to be more effective than methotrexate in patients with early RA in a 12-month trial.

Infliximab is a chimeric (part-mouse, part-human) mAb to TNF-α, administered by intravenous infusion (Figure 9.2). Infliximab has also been shown in placebo-controlled trials to reduce inflammatory activity

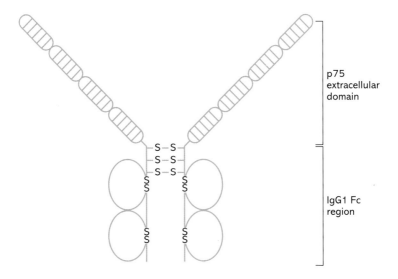

Figure 9.1 Etanercept structure. S–S indicates disulphide bridges.

and improve quality of life and, in combination with methotrexate, to inhibit radiographic disease progression. Interestingly, radiographic progression was slowed even in patients who did not appear to respond clinically with a reduction in joint inflammation. Co-administration of methotrexate with infliximab significantly reduces the formation of antibodies directed against the murine portion of the molecule, which would otherwise neutralize its efficacy. Infliximab is currently recommended for use only with concomitant methotrexate therapy, at an initial dose of 3 mg/kg every 8 weeks.

Characteristics of TNF inhibitors. In addition to improvements in inflammation and joint damage, patients receiving TNF-α inhibitors also report important reductions in fatigue and malaise. This is a unique feature of these therapies and provides important quality-of-life benefits. Aside from differences in immunogenicity, half-life, and route of administration, there are additional theoretical differences between etanercept and infliximab. For example, etanercept also neutralizes TNF-β (lymphotoxin), although the contribution of this feature to efficacy or toxicity is uncertain.

Novel TNF-α antagonists are in development and a number are currently undergoing phase II and III trials. These include a fully humanized anti-TNF-α mAb, and a p55 TNF receptor dimer containing a polyethylene glycol linker.

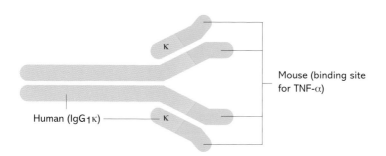

Figure 9.2 Infliximab is a chimeric antibody; mouse sequence is shown in green, human in orange.

For uncertain reasons, not all RA patients respond to TNF-α antagonists, and at present there are no factors that can be used to predict efficacy. Additionally, long-term follow-up is required of patients treated with these therapies before we will know their exact place in the treatment of RA.

Post-marketing surveillance has led to the recognition of certain uncommon adverse effects of TNF-α blockade. These include the reactivation of dormant tuberculosis, and episodes of central nervous system demyelination.

Interleukin-1 antagonism

The role of IL-1 in the pathogenesis of RA is reviewed in Chapter 3. In particular, IL-1 is thought to play a major pro-inflammatory role in RA, but also to be an important stimulus to erosion development and bone destruction. The successful use of neutralizing anti-IL-1 antibodies in animal models of arthritis has demonstrated the involvement of IL-1β in the development and progression of arthritis in mice.

IL-1 receptor antagonist (IL-1ra) and soluble IL-1 receptors (sIL-1Rs) are natural inhibitors of IL-1 and are produced locally at sites of inflammation. In RA, however, there appears to be an imbalance that favours the pro-inflammatory actions of IL-1. An attractive approach to the treatment of inflammatory diseases is therefore the use of recombinant IL-1ra (rIL-1ra) (Figure 9.3) or recombinant sIL-1Rs (rhusIL-1Rs) (Figure 9.4) to shift the balance toward an anti-inflammatory state.

In a placebo-controlled, double-blind study, 472 RA patients were given either IL-1ra (at doses of 30, 75 or 150 mg/day) or placebo by daily subcutaneous injection for 24 weeks. A significant number of patients receiving high-dose IL-1ra achieved ACR20 response criteria (see page 60). Acute-phase reactant levels – erythrocyte sedimentation rate (ESR) and C-reactive protein (CRP) – improved, and there was evidence of slowing of progressive joint-space narrowing and slowing in the rate of joint erosions. The combination of IL-1ra and methotrexate has also been shown to be more effective than methotrexate alone.

IL-1ra (anakinra) is generally well tolerated. Mild transient injection-site reactions have been the most common adverse events reported.

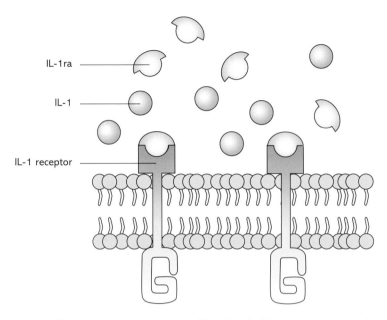

IL-1ra

IL-1

IL-1 receptor

Figure 9.3 Diagrammatic representation of how interleukin-1 receptor antagonist (IL-1ra) inhibits activities of IL-1.

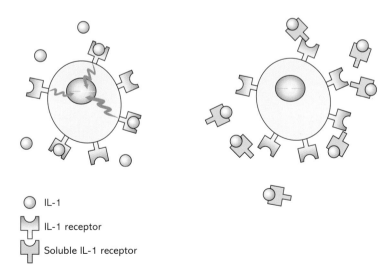

○ IL-1

IL-1 receptor

Soluble IL-1 receptor

Figure 9.4 Diagrammatic representation of how soluble receptors bind to circulating interleukin-1 (IL-1) and inhibit its activity.

83

> **Key points**
>
> - TNF-α blockade and IL-1 receptor antagonism are now 'in the clinic'.
> - Both types of therapy slow joint damage more effectively than traditional DMARDs.
> - These are expensive, 'biologically produced' drugs that require parenteral (intravenous or subcutaneous) administration.
> - Not all patients respond to these therapies, presumably reflecting important interpatient differences in disease pathogenesis.
> - Prolonged experience with these drugs will be required to provide a true therapeutic ratio and accurate economic evaluation.

Anakinra was approved by the US FDA in November 2001 and by the EMEA in March 2002.

Conclusions regarding biological response modifiers

TNF inhibitors have provided a major advance in our therapeutic options for treating RA. Understanding why some patients do not respond to these therapies remains a challenge and provides opportunities for a better understanding of the pathogenetic mechanisms operative in RA. With the advent of IL-1 antagonists, clinicians may soon be able to provide a combination of targeted therapies (combined TNF-α and IL-1 inhibitors) that block different aspects of the pathological process in RA. Important questions that remain regarding these therapies include the likelihood of opportunistic or unusual infections in the context of their chronic administration. It also remains to be determined whether chronic TNF-α blockade will result in an increased incidence of tumours. Finally, the costs of these potent biological therapies will need to be evaluated in terms of their long-term benefit, with particular regard to work stability, the predicted reduction in joint replacements, and their potential to provide improved quality of life and lifespan (see Chapter 4). The question whether

TNF-α- or IL-1-inhibitors should or will replace methotrexate or sulfasalazine as the DMARDs of first choice will be answered only as the use of these agents increases. In the UK, NICE guidance, issued in March 2002, suggests the use of a TNF-α inhibitor only in patients with active RA who have not responded adequately to at least two DMARDs, including methotrexate (unless contraindicated). Therapy should only be undertaken by a consultant rheumatologist with monitoring of the DAS28 score (see page 61) as a measure of efficacy. The latter recommendations have been issued by the British Society for Rheumatology, who also run a centralized database for all patients receiving BRMs. At present in the USA the use of TNF-α- or IL-1-inhibitors is reserved for patients who have had an incomplete or inadequate response to DMARDs, such as methotrexate. Clinical trials being conducted will help to address critical issues as to when in the course of disease these agents might best be used alone or in combination.

Key references

Bathon JM, Martin RW, Fleischmann RM et al. A comparison of etanercept and methotrexate in patients with early rheumatoid arthritis. N Engl J Med 2000;343: 1586–93.

Bresnihan B, Alvaro-Gracia JM, Cobby M et al. Treatment of rheumatoid arthritis with recombinant human interleukin-1 receptor antagonist. Arthritis Rheum 1998;41:2196–204.

Lipsky PE, van der Heijde DM, St Clair EW et al. Infliximab and methotrexate in the treatment of rheumatoid arthritis. Anti-Tumor Necrosis Factor Trial in Rheumatoid Arthritis with Concomitant Therapy Study Group. N Engl J Med 2000;343:1594–602.

Maini RN, Breedveld FC, Kalden JR et al. Therapeutic efficacy of multiple intravenous infusions of anti-tumor necrosis factor alpha monoclonal antibody combined with low-dose weekly methotrexate in rheumatoid arthritis. Arthritis Rheum 1998;41:1552–63.

Moreland LW, Baumgartner SW, Schiff MH *et al*. Treatment of rheumatoid arthritis with a recombinant human tumor necrosis factor receptor (p75)-Fc fusion protein. *N Engl J Med* 1997;337: 141–7.

Weinblatt ME, Kremer JM, Bankhurst AD *et al*. A trial of etanercept, a recombinant tumor necrosis factor receptor: Fc fusion protein, in patients with rheumatoid arthritis receiving methotrexate. *N Engl J Med* 1999;340:253–9.

Biological therapy

Numerous potential targets for BRMs are currently under investigation. Those that are showing the most promise include co-stimulation blockers and mitogen-activated protein kinase (MAPK) inhibitors.

Blocking of co-stimulation. Several biological agents directed against co-stimulatory molecules (or their ligands) have been tested in animal models of autoimmune disease and may be clinically useful in humans. In addition to interaction of the T-cell receptor with its peptide-MHC ligand, a succession of secondary, or co-stimulatory, molecular interactions are required for full T-cell activation. The main second signal is provided by interaction of CD28 on the T-cell with B7.1 (CD80) and B7.2 (CD86) on the antigen-presenting cell (APC). CD40 on the APC also interacts with CD40 ligand (CD40L or CD154, a member of the TNF family of proteins) on the T-cell, providing additional signals. Following activation, cytotoxic T-lymphocyte associated protein 4 (CTLA 4, CD152) is upregulated on the T-cell. This is a downregulatory molecule that has a 100-fold higher affinity for CD80 and CD86 than does CD28, and contributes to the cessation of the immune response.

Potential cellular targets for immunotherapy in humans therefore include CD40, CD40 ligand, CD80, CD86 and CD28 (Figure 10.1). Clinical trials are currently underway in RA of a fusion protein consisting of the extracellular portion of CTLA 4 and the Fc portion of human IgG1 (CTLA4-Ig), which prevents binding of B7 to CD28. In a phase I study in patients with psoriasis, CTLA4-Ig treatment resulted in a 50% or greater improvement in clinical disease activity, with clinical improvements showing a dose–response relationship. Blockade of the CD40/CD40L interaction has also been attempted in patients with systemic lupus erythematosus.

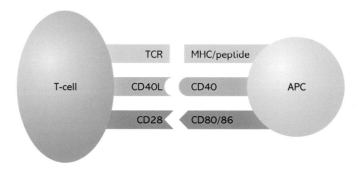

Figure 10.1 A few of the critical cell surface interactions between a T-cell and an antigen-presenting cell.

Signal transmission inhibition. Inflammatory and destructive responses require appropriate gene activation. In turn, these genes are activated through cascades of signalling molecules. In immune and inflammatory cells, important signalling molecules include nuclear factor-kappa B (NF-κB) and the MAPKs (sometimes called stress kinases). Expression of these molecules is modified in response to physical stresses and inflammatory triggers such as cytokines, fever, shock, ischaemia or toxins. The targeting of these molecules therefore provides an attractive therapeutic strategy in RA. Theoretically, blockade of appropriate signalling pathways could downregulate genes critical not only for inflammation but also for synoviocyte proliferation and cartilage and bone destruction. P38 is a particular MAPK and is believed to upregulate TNF-α, IL-1, IL-6, IL-8 and nitric oxide production, and COX-2 expression. P38 MAPK inhibitors have been shown to be efficacious in several disease models, including inflammation, septic shock, and animal models of arthritis. Several p38 MAPK inhibitors are under investigation in man for the treatment of autoimmune-based disease. Not only do these agents offer the potential to modulate a variety of unwanted cellular responses but they are also active when given orally.

Gene therapy

Some of the BRMs, such as IL-1ra and other cytokine-based therapies, are limited by an extremely short half-life. Gene therapy provides a potential means of overcoming the requirement for daily injections. Essentially, the gene encoding the therapeutic product is inserted into a non-replicative viral vector. This is then used to introduce the gene into a recipient either systemically via the bloodstream, or locally into tissues. A number of examples have been successfully applied to animal models of arthritis, and phase I studies in osteoarthritis have been performed in Pittsburgh. The main limitations at present are generalized safety issues relating to the use of viral vectors, and the need to identify robust methods for regulating transcription and translation of the therapeutic gene.

Genetics

The sequencing of the human genome has provided a more or less complete list of genes that can be translated into protein products. Many were previously identified but a significant number are novel. Powerful techniques now exist to compare the transcription of tens of thousands of these genes between different tissues. Such analyses are being used to study different types of arthritic synovium. Such work should provide novel insights into disease pathogenesis as well as additional therapeutic avenues and prognostic markers.

Similar approaches applied to genomic DNA prepared from blood can provide a genetic fingerprint of the individual, highlighting the presence or absence of polymorphisms in a variety of genes. Such analyses might ultimately be used to predict the susceptibility of an individual to RA. In the individual with established disease, it should become possible to predict responsiveness to specific drugs. This science is termed pharmacogenetics and offers the promise of initiating drugs with predicted efficacy at disease onset.

Advances in surgery

Although reconstructive surgery has been one of the major advances for improving the quality of life of many RA patients, there are limitations including loosening of the prosthetic joints and inadequate prosthetic replacements for several joints (e.g. ankle, shoulder). A large body of knowledge is accumulating concerning prosthetic joint loosening, which should result in the development of techniques and strategies to prolong the life of artificial joints. Furthermore, progress is being made in the design and implementation of novel joint prostheses.

Newer imaging modalities

MRI and HRUS (see Chapter 6) are becoming routinely available in some centres in Europe, providing high-resolution and three-dimensional images of the inflamed joint and surrounding structures. Recent advances include the incorporation of Doppler into musculoskeletal ultrasound probes, enabling an estimation of blood flow in addition to structural information. Newer MRI magnets are now available for the study of peripheral joints, which provide high-resolution images of, for example, the hand and wrist, without the limitations imposed by the use of whole-body magnets.

Stem cell biology

The identification of mesenchymal stem cells has offered hope that defects in cartilage and bone can be repaired by autologous chondrocyte or osteoblast precursors in an appropriate matrix. Although such technology is likely to be applied initially to osteoarthritic joints, a role in RA may become evident, particularly if mesenchymal defects are shown to play a primary role in disease pathogenesis.

Key references

Abrams JR, Lebwohl MG, Guzzo CA et al. CTLA4Ig-mediated blockade of T-cell costimulation in patients with psoriasis vulgaris. J Clin Invest 1999;103:1243–1252.

CH Evans, SC Ghivizzani, R Kang et al. Gene therapy for rheumatic diseases. Arthritis Rheum 1999; 42:1–16.

Koopman WJ. Prospects for autoimmune disease: research advances in rheumatoid arthritis. JAMA 2001; 285:648–650.

McGonagle D, Conaghan PG, Wakefield R, Emery P. Imaging the joints in early rheumatoid arthritis. Best Pract Res Clin Rheumatol 201;15:91–104.

Useful addresses

American College of Rheumatology
1800 Century Place, Suite 250
Atlanta, GA 30345-4300, USA
phone: 404 633 3777
fax: 404 633 1870
acr@rheumatology.org
www.rheumatology.org
[Rheumatologists' association]

Arthritis Care
18 Stephenson Way
London NW1 2HD, UK
phone: 020 7380 6500
fax: 020 7380 6505
helpline: 080 8800 4050
(free, weekdays 12:00–16:00)
thesource@arthritiscare.org.uk
www.arthritiscare.org.uk
[Patient support group (e-mail address is
for young people with arthritis)]

Arthritis Foundation
PO Box 7669
Atlanta, GA 30357-0669, USA
phone: 1 800 283 7800
www.arthritis.org
[Patient support group]

Arthritis Research Campaign
St Mary's Court, St Mary's Gate
Chesterfield, Derbyshire S41 7TD, UK
phone: 01246 558033
fax: 01246 558007
info@arc.org.uk
www.arc.org.uk
[Charity funding rheumatology research
and patient support]

British Society for Rheumatology
41 Eagle Street
London WC1R 4TL
phone: 020 7242 3313
fax: 020 7242 3277
bsr@rheumatology.org.uk
www.rheumatology.org.uk
[Rheumatologists' association]

European League Against Rheumatism
Eular Secretariat
Witikonerstrasse 15
CH-8032 Zurich
Switzerland
phone: 01383 9690
fax: 01383 9810
eular@bluewin.ch
www.eular.org
[Rheumatologists' association]

International League of Associations for
Rheumatology
www.ilar.org

Primary Care Rheumatology Society
PO Box 42, Northallerton
North Yorkshire DL7 8YG
phone: 01609 774974
fax: 01609 774726
helen@pcrsociety.freeserve.co.uk
info@pcrsociety.com
www.pcrsociety.com
[General practitioners interested in
rheumatology]

Index